Dance like the stars.

*The philosophy of physical expression,
the learning process & celebrity fitness…*

By Anthony King

A TICK TICK MEDIA PAPERBACK

First published in Great Britain in 2007 by

Tick Tick Media
Flat 318
456-458 Strand
Trafalgar Square
London
WC2R 0DZ

Copyright @ Anthony King 2007

The right of Anthony King to be identified as the author of this work has been asserted to him in accordance with the Copyright, Designs and Patents Act 1988

All rights reserved. No part of this publication may be reproduced, stored in a retrieval system, or transmitted, in any form or by any means, electronic, mechanical, photocopying, recording or otherwise, without the prior permission of the copyright owner.

A CIP catalogue record for this book is available from the British Library

ISBN 978-0-9555788-0-9

Design/artwork and illustrations by Shivraj Gohil
Photography by Dash Gohil

To Ryan, Sidney and my dearest brother Westley

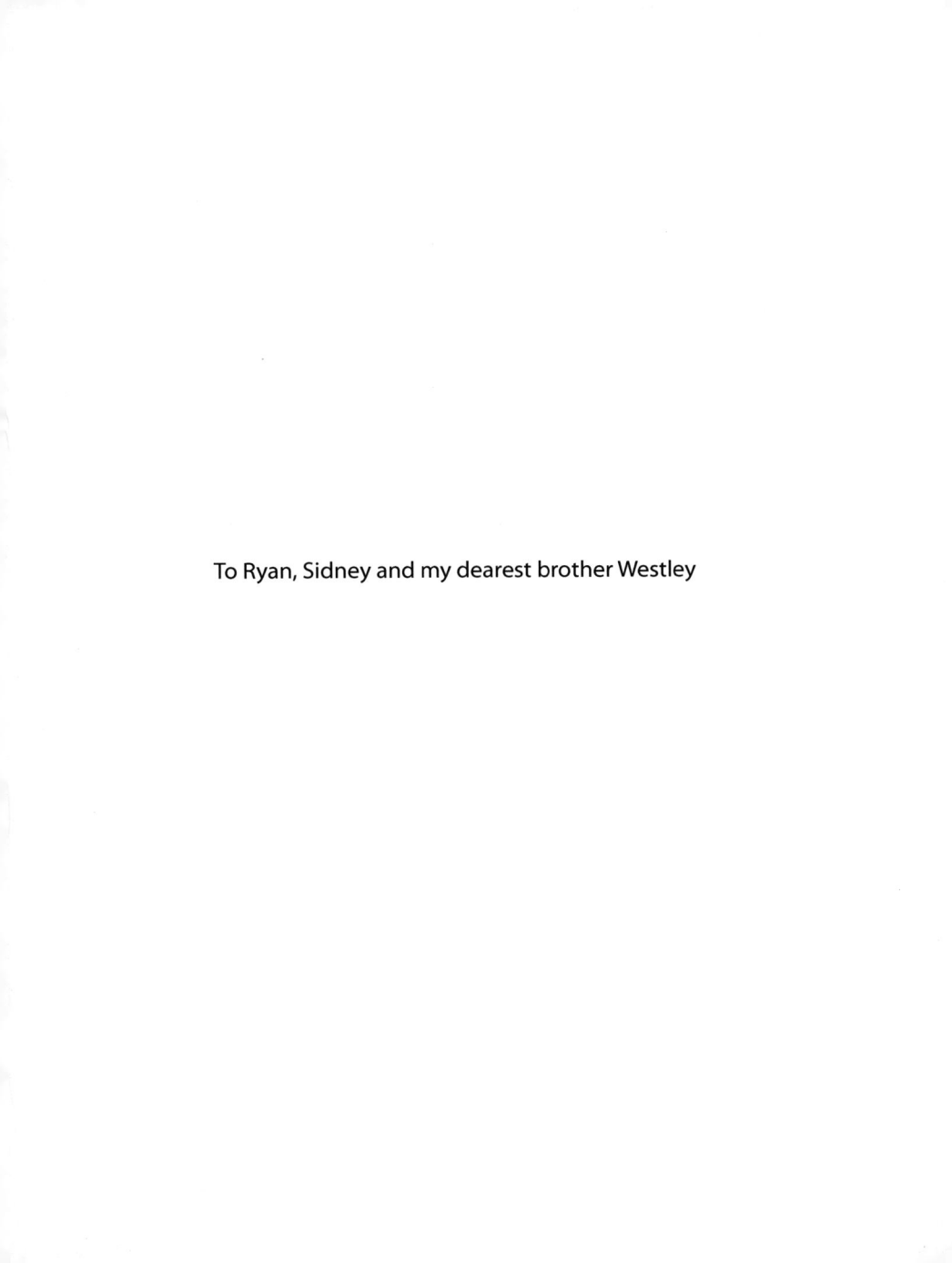

Disclaimer

It is advisable to consult a physician in all matters relating to health and in particular to check with your doctor before embarking on any exercise regime. While the advice and information in this book is believed to be accurate and true at the time of going to press, neither the author nor the publisher can accept any legal responsibility or liability for any injury sustained whilst following the exercises or advice.

Contents

Part 1: A closer look at ourselves: The learning process

Preface	5
Introduction	17
Self perspective	24
What makes you unique?	29
Psychological Projection	31
Determining what's possible and impossible for you	33
The experts get it wrong!	36
Why you should dance, if that's what you want	43
Can we learn from the attitude of our children?	51
How to feel great and have fun!	57

Part 2: Celebrity Fitness

You are what you eat	77
A simple and healthy framework	79
Different types of Carbohydrates	82
Fibre	85
Your energy level and the Glycaemic index	86

Your body's Insulin level	90
Carbohydrates and well being	92
Proteins	93
Healthy Amino Acids	95
Protein and how it affects your mood	96
Fats	99
Important Fatty Acids	101
How to feel energized!	104
Water, Food, Exercise and Sleep	106
Healthy eating	109
What should we eat?	111
General Fitness	113
Feeling great!	114
Ways of becoming more active	115
Easy ways of boosting your metabolism	116
Dance and Aerobic fitness	117

Part 3: Dance and physical expression

Capturing the beauty of nature to enhance your dance and movement aesthetically	120
What makes a "good" dance move "good" and a "bad" dance move "bad"?	121
What is "Divine proportion" and how does it relate to dance and movement?	124
What exactly is "dance" and how do I improve it?	138
Poise	142
Style	143
Timing	144
Control	146
Placement & Accuracy	147
Learning the Moonwalk!	148
The side slide!	155
Simple Stretching	166
Some fun ways to keep toned	171
Conclusion	174
Acknowledgments	177
Bibliography	180

Preface

I've always asked myself when looking at great artists perform or at an amazing piece of art, music or architecture, what is it that makes it or them so special? What is it that differentiates that person from the rest? Do they have a supernatural ability or a connection to something greater that we will never know? Or is it a talent that can be learnt? When we see a painting by Leonardo Da Vinci or hear an amazing piece of music by Beethoven, we see and hear near perfection that leaves us awestruck, but where does the magic that we all recognise as genius come from? Could it be a particular age or demographic? It would seem that it's something more than learning a particular skill and practising a lot. The magic comes from the unique individual, the magic flows through them and it is they who are the key to unlocking that potential. They possess a particular mindset or belief and a unique way of looking at themselves and the world…

So before a musical note, a dance step or any kind of conceivable expression is executed physically in the world, it is firstly an expression of who you are mentally, spiritually and physically. The physical execution, although essential, is last in the chain and it is the physical action that is the easiest to replicate and duplicate. The other parts take some understanding, effort and thought. For example, before carrying out the execution of a dance step it is of utmost importance that we understand our own intentions so that we can then convey that step effectively to others to appreciate and admire in physical form.

It's the great artists that execute a step or the mesmerising singer who hits the right note who understand that a physical act is by no means the whole story! I'm talking about passion, belief and understanding. Of course with training and repetition you can program somebody to physically move in a certain way. However, there will always be the exceptional few that have something extra…that magic that is clear to see.

This is something that is missing from the solely physical thinking person who may believe that by schooling alone you can master your craft. I'm talking about the difference between a *true dancer* and somebody that can move their body. I'm talking about the lasting artist who inspires and gives hope as opposed to one who entertains briefly and is soon forgotten. There is a big difference. The difference is down to the artist: who they are, how they think and what they stand for.

An artist is an artist all of the time. A star is born a star (It's just a case of rediscovering who you really are) understanding yourself and working hard to perfect your skill, whatever that may be. It is an essential for all artists. So before you start on that journey it makes sense to think about who you are, what you stand for and how you can best be yourself. After that it's simply a case of just letting the magic flow through you…

"Dance like the stars- Book 1", is essentially a combination of articles and blog posts that I wrote during the latter part of 2006. My primary aim was for the book to serve as an accompaniment for any artistic thinking person, in the psychological processes of physical expression. As well as, how to think like an artist and a unique person. Dancing is just a physical expression of who you are and if you want to become a better dancer or a better thinker, the rules are the same through every area of your life.

Ranging from Individuality, to Self perspective, to the execution of a precise dance step, I have started, with Book 1, to look at what I believe are the most important aspects of true artistic expression. Firstly trying to understand who we are as individuals as well as artists and secondly how to convey who we are to others through the physical movement of our body. After thinking about our mental processes and trying to understand who we are, it's important not to forget that we convey this through our physical body! A large part of this first book takes a look at nutrition and health so that we can all perform to our optimum level.

My primary aim, through this book is to encourage you to think about yourself as an individual and the way in which you express yourself to the world. Not to teach you to dance or to teach you anything at all - just for you to think about yourself and where you are going, and possibly give you a little encouragement to trust in yourself and express yourself in your own unique way. Do with this book as you please, as it's yours after all. Take your marker and highlight portions, skip the health bits if you want. Start at the back and work forwards even! You are free to pick and choose whatever bits you feel are relevant and helpful for you just as you are free to try something new and to finally get working on yourself, your goals and your dreams...It is *never* too late for that.

The ancients, while navigating the high seas used to look to the stars for guidance and direction. They would use the constellations to plot their course through the rough seas and stormy weather. Even with clouds and pouring rain, hope would return with the clear skies and with it clear direction, renewed hope and safety. Likewise, the ancient Egyptians, who influenced the world we live in beyond measure, were highly proficient in computing the power of the planets, luminaries and constellations and the interactions between them. As they looked up, they believed, as did the Greeks and civilisations before them that it was these heavenly bodies which had an effect upon the destinies of nations as well as individuals. It was the stars they looked up to and regarded as living things that influenced us. Today, we still look up to the "stars" for guidance, fashion tips, and inspiration. Pop stars, "Superstars" and so called "talented" people, seemingly unreachable up on the Billboards and on television – out of our grasp. People placed in positions, adored and ready to be knocked down or carted off to rehab. It's amazing how much power and influence the few wield over the masses. Pythagoras himself, the first "Philosopher" considered "the stars" to be "bodies" that encased souls, minds and spirits. It is quite clear that today as we look up to our own "pop idols", the latest marketed talents and stars we should ask ourselves, are they really worthy of being emulated and adored? Should we not instead focus our energies on expressing ourselves to the best of our own abilities? Surely this is far healthier than trying to complete a near-impossible task and mimic those who we place up on the mantle piece ready, at any point to be knocked down, revealing themselves to be just as infallible as the rest of us?

These are not only philosophical questions but are most relevant for the artists, dancers, actors, musicians and entertainers among us - the true artists that will at least strive to be the best that they can be. The artists that dig deeper. Those who understand it is harmony that is a prerequisite of beauty. That the beautiful poem, dance, song, piece of music or expression is only so when its parts are harmonious. The message is clear; you will have to search for yourself, your self if you want to find that harmonious combination that will raise YOU up to the next level as an artist and a person. Search. You. For yourself.

Some might ask, what has philosophy and self knowledge got to do with modern pop culture and practical advancement of their dancing, singing, acting, song writing and performing? I would say that anybody who asks that question is not ready for the answer, as it would be of no use to them. Instead of turning on the television or immersing oneself in temporary pop culture for inspiration and direction, would it not make sense at least to take a look at the real teachers who created the whole system that we live in today?

Budding musicians and serious songwriters might, for example, find out who exactly is credited with the discovery of the diatonic scale, the foundation of every piece of music that we listen to. Who was it that coined the word "tone"? Who pondered upon the laws of consonance and dissonance for years? Who understood and explained them? They might discover who first understood and explained the amazing and often overwhelming effect of sound and music on the senses and our emotional state, i.e. music and its power to influence the mind and body. It is clear that even the modern greats like Madonna, Michael Jackson or Paul McCartney are not going to give you a blank stare if you talk about the details of their craft, because they understand the importance of knowledge - and if you want to be as great as them, then you should be looking in that direction too. They would know how the Druids used melody to heal, as they believed it soothed the physical body as well as the soul. How they also believed that the strings of their harps were tuned to the planets and why.

This in turn, might be of interest to the curious actor or student of English and Drama. Especially one that has read "The Merchant of Venice", for example. A different perspective on what the author actually meant when writing; "There's not the smallest orb which thou behold'st but in his motion like an angel sings". That same line of the Shakespearian play might become even more interesting to the theologian when we look toward the reference works and the words of "Job" when he described a time "when the stars of the morning sang together". It is quite clear: art, music, philosophy, theology and culture are all linked and the true artist should learn from them all - but let's leave that for another day and look toward dance right now!

So don't forget: YOU are an individual. Follow your *own* path and your own dreams, of your own choosing! Always ask questions. Search for your own truth. Express yourself in as unique a way as possible. I'll leave you with the wisest words that I have ever heard from a teacher - the words of the first philosopher Pythagoras: "Know thyself"

Anthony King
London, England
March 15, 2007

Introduction

Welcome! My name is Anthony King, I'm a choreographer and a dance teacher. As you're reading this I'm going to assume that you want to improve your dancing abilities and build your confidence! Don't worry - I'm going to show you how you can achieve this for yourself whilst revealing who you really are inside.

You might have always dreamed of being the person who's in the middle of the dance floor, whom everybody looks at and says "Wow, they're amazing!" Or maybe you just long for the ability to impress your friends and family with a classic step or two. Maybe, deep in your heart you just want the ability to walk into a club and be comfortable to be yourself and not have to stand in the corner with your drink watching everybody else having fun. Hey, maybe you think that you look like a fool on the move when you dance and you want to change that! No problem. I'm here to tell you right now, that it is more than possible and you can have more than that! If you want to, you can dance like the stars!

I've taught thousands of people from all over the world, from the absolute beginner to the professional dancer. I've learned that when it comes to dance, it doesn't matter what demographic you fit into. Whatever your race, age, size or ability, we all have the same fears to overcome, and most importantly, with a little effort, we all have the ability to overcome them. I'm talking about the investment banker, who always dreamed of dancing, but took the "sensible" route into the corporate world, to the school teacher who feels the same. I've taught people from all walks of life, from millionaires who want to do something different, to some big stars who want to learn an exciting new piece of choreography or absolute beginners who want to learn a step or two, for work or fun!

A while back I was on the phone to a member of world renowned rock group "Pink Floyd" who have sold over 100 million albums. We were discussing some special choreography for a show; I'm going to tell you exactly what I told him, "If you really want to do it…we can do it, no problem, that's your choice, but you have to be in 100%. It's really nothing to do with me, it's up to you…but if you're serious then we can do it". He agreed, with a chuckle, and I hope you do to! It is your choice! (The smile and chuckle bit is the most important!). Dancing is largely about fun in the first place! I'll be honest with you, and let you into a little secret, you probably don't need me to teach you to dance. No, that wasn't a mistake: you probably don't need me to teach you to dance! The art of dancing is not an external thing that you learn "out there" in the world. There are some very special unique exceptions (medical for example), but generally it's not something that needs to be taught or learned. Can I teach you a step, or a move, or a piece of choreography? Yes, of course I can, but to dance, to dance is to be yourself, the person that you really are inside. You are a creature of rhythm! You may think that you haven't got any rhythm but that's the point, you *think* that you haven't got any rhythm and that my friend is an incorrect thought!

Dancing well is a state of oneness, of being you and having fun! The most important thing to remember is to lose your inhibitions. When dancing, fear can be the big negative force which can imprison you and hold you back. Fear is not a physical issue, it is a mental barrier, which we usually create ourselves (however let's put this aside for now and deal with it later). The bottom line is that dance is a mental expression of who and what you are and secondly, it is a physical expression and manifestation of how you feel. That's all well and good I hear you say, "I'll just imagine that I'm Michael Jackson, or Madonna, or Justin Timberlake and then I'll go out and dance like them…yeah right….you haven't see me dance!" indeed, you would have a point! It's only the first logical step, but it is a first step that can't be missed or skipped.

There's no denying that results require a combination of actions and thoughts, along with practice and logical hard work – these are key. Different action equals different result. Same action equals same result. It's important though, that you think about each step separately before moving on. I'm talking about walking into a dance class and sneaking out, because you're scared or hiding at the back, or "joke" dancing, where you pretend you don't care but really do, or staring through the window, wishing. Those days are over! As the scientist Albert Einstein said, "Insanity: doing the same thing over and over again and expecting different results". If you've always been too scared to apply yourself, or are always stuck behind those four or five amazing dancers at the front of class, or didn't even have the courage to make it out of your bedroom or the moves in the living room: then let's start afresh. Think logically and truthfully, by taking a closer look at ourselves and our own thought processes. We will have a much better chance of getting positive results.

Now, some good news: however bad you think you are there is always somebody worse! That's a joke, but it has indeed got an element of truth in it. The point being that we do not have the ability as humans to judge ourselves in an objective and fair way. So it doesn't matter how badly (or well for that matter!) you may think you dance; you're probably not the best judge either way and you're probably a lot better than you are able to see or acknowledge. The French author Anais Nin put it this way; "We don't see things as they are. We see them as we are". In my opinion she was right. I also think *that* alone is the key to any expressive act and any expression of who you are. Remember that movement and dance are just expressions of who you are to the beat of drum, nothing more, nothing less.

Dance and movement are mental expressions of who you are in a physical manifestation. Let's take an example; a young Lawyer (let's call him Tom) walks into a club with his friends and after a few drinks decides that he is "the man" and that he is going to impress the ladies on the other side of the dance floor with some "cool moves". Tom wants to impress them, he's showing off and he wants to get their attention. When he finally hits the dance floor, he feels that everybody is looking at him and decides to really go for it; he sees people smiling and decides to add a little bit more energy and spice it up with a bit of comedy too! Now he really has the girls' attention, in fact they're almost in tears from all the laughter. So the young Lawyer responds in turn with laughter and a cheeky smile, returning to his group of friends for the "high fives" and more alcohol. Although this seems funny, and "a good laugh", it wasn't really the reaction that Tom was honestly looking for, and although the reaction to his "performance", was a joy to behold, it was a joy for everybody else. That joy doesn't trickle down to him, because deep down, he really wanted to dance and look natural and be himself and not just the court jester. So Tom, smiles and jests with his pals, it seems great and everybody's happy! But wait a second....something is amiss. Well, deep down in Tom's heart, although it was a laugh, he doesn't feel so good about it. He earns £100,000 a year, he's a "success", a great lawyer, in fact he's the best. Tom is not a court joker and doesn't really appreciate the reaction he got. In fact he's really upset about it, but tomorrow's another day and life goes on….let's have another drink! Tomorrow he'll be at work and he'll be the star!

It's always the same story. The person who sees everybody else dancing amazingly, having so much fun, and the feeling of being left out. The feeling that *I* could never do that. It is not possible for me to be that good or that cool or that hip. It just isn't possible on this planet.

Let's take a look at the problem

Straight off the bat, we've already established that we're not accurate at judging ourselves in an objective way. So a message for anybody who thinks that they "can't dance" or don't have any "rhythm": your premise is wrong and that's why you come to the incorrect conclusion that you don't have the ability or can't dance. It is the thought process which is flawed NOT you or your ability. In a moment I'm going to show you why you're wrong if you think that you haven't got any rhythm but before I do, let's take a closer look at "Self Perspective".

False self perspective is probably the biggest dream killer. If you're going to abandon or give up on an ambition, goal or lifelong dream, then let it be based upon a true reflection of your ability, rather than a lie or an incorrectly held opinion of yourself as dictated or influenced by others.

Self Perspective

Let's be realistic about all this "positive" thinking for a moment:

Question:

If I simply think that I can dance like Michael Jackson or the famous ballerina Alicia Alonso, does that mean that I can dance like them straight away?

Answer:

No, of course not! (You're having a laugh!)

…but that's not the question we should be asking. A more appropriate question might be:

Question:

If I have a negative self perspective of myself or my abilities, can this fact impede my development and progress, regardless of my actual ability or the truth of the matter?

Answer:

Yes. Absolutely!

The main factor to consider is "negative" self perspective and thinking, and more importantly, *incorrect* negative thinking! That is the killer that will prevent your progress in any field at all: false self perspective is probably the biggest dream killer there is and it's the saddest! If you're going to abandon or give up on an ambition, goal or lifelong dream, then let it be based upon a true reflection of your ability and contributing factors rather than a lie or an incorrectly held opinion of yourself as dictated or influenced by others! And yes, we are all influenced by outside factors which we usually give merit and weight to undeservedly. Sometimes we take the word and opinions of others over and above that of our own. Is it possible that we alone are the ones who ultimately know what's good for us and our personal limitations?

…I would say yes! Remember, things can change, and experts can be wrong too!

You alone are the best judge of your potential abilities!

You alone are the best judge of your potential abilities. Why? Because only you know how far you are willing to go to do something or what kind of real commitment and sacrifice you're willing to give to attaining a goal. In fact you are the number one expert in the field of you! You will always have the edge because only you know what's going on inside and the depth of your passion. The truth and the key to unlocking your true potential lie inside you alone. We all know the difference between right and wrong (and the bottom line as to whether something is really possible or not) if we've cheated at something, if we did the right thing or wrong thing. You can just look in the mirror. The truth is instinctively hot wired into us. We don't need an expert or a teacher to enlighten us - although we might need a gentle reminder at times to reinforce the truth that we already know, deep down inside. My high school drama teacher, Mr Oades, reminded me one day after class "Anthony, in the quiet times, when we look inside ourselves, we all know the truth".

So:

- Can I really learn to dance?
- Can I run the London Marathon?
- Am I able to learn to play the piano?
- Is it possible to lose weight?
- Can I pass this exam?
- Can I get a degree?
- Can I achieve my dreams?
- Will I ever be in control of my own destiny?

Answer:

Only you know for sure: You are the number one expert in the field of you!

I know for sure that if you really chose to achieve any one of your goals you could achieve it. At the end of the day what would stop you? If you made the ultimate conscious decision then you would find a way to over come any barrier, or if you don't have the resources you might work a way around them or change the rules. Remember there is no fixed script or perfect map for achieving anything. Rewrite the rules, redefine boundaries as you go. You are free to do what you want and that is part of the fun. The creative genius Paul Arden put it this way, "you may have to beg, steal and borrow to get it done. But that's for you to work out how to do it". The bottom line…

The parameters of your goal or dream should only be defined by its author…you!

We often allow others to define our goals and dreams and sometimes, even our lives. We came into this world as unique individuals and it's my opinion that there is no better feeling than being yourself and making your own decisions! It's one of the biggest tragedies to lose that individuality and uniqueness by letting it be moulded by the world around you, by allowing it to supersede your own opinions, thoughts and desires. Let's take a closer look at individuality and uniqueness.

"Most people are other people. Their thoughts are someone else's opinions, their lives a mimicry, their passions a quotation"
Oscar Wilde

Am I an Individual? What makes me unique?

Am I an individual? What makes *me* unique? Do I even have the ability to answer the question? I think that we all like to *think* of ourselves as unique people and we surely hope that we are, but what's the fact of the matter? What makes me different from the next person? The writer Alan Watts points out something very interesting:

"We seldom realize, for example, that our most private thoughts and emotions are not actually our own. For we think in terms of languages and images which we did not invent, but which were given to us by our society. We copy emotional parents… society is our extended mind and body"

So, Alan Watts is saying that we copy our emotional responses from our parents. So is it possible that even that which we claim to be our inner thoughts and opinions didn't really originate from us? Now that's a thought! If they didn't originate uniquely from us and were possibly placed upon us, then what hope would we have for style, talent or anything else! Let's take a look at that though. We are trained beings, we do what our parents and teachers taught us, turning us into what we are today. We are bombarded daily with what we need to buy or think or consume, in order that we may be happy or popular. We are engulfed with the concepts of what our limitations are and our "place" in society. The idea that we will never be like those amazing people "up there" in front of the bright lights and walking down the red carpets on TV or in the movies and magazines, constantly. This as though those people are from another planet, different from the rest of us. That's just what is thrust on us from the billboards and advertisements on a walk down any road, daily. We are being spoken to, literally all the time through advertising, TV and the media, parents and friends, colleagues etc.

Does the world influence you? Does it enhance your uniqueness, buying into somebody else's idea of beauty, success or morals, or does it detract from you?

Hmmm…..so when I say to myself "I'll never be able to dance like that!" Am I being fair? Am I being honest or am I just repeating what I think to be correct because I'm not thinking "outside the box", but inside the parameters set by other people (which are usually so limiting)? I would say that it's based on other people projecting onto you and you reflecting that back.

The key points to remember are that

- You are the number one expert
- You define your own parameters
- What's good for everybody else might not and probably isn't perfect for you or your set of unique talents and set of circumstances.

A closer look at: Psychological Projection

"We project our own unpleasant feelings onto someone else and blame them for having thoughts that we really have."

Put simply, this is somebody telling you, for example,

"You'll never go far"

Or

"That's a really competitive field. Do you really want to risk it?"

Or

"Are you really going to wear that dress?"

When somebody restricts you or tells you that you can't do something, or has such negative opinions of your chances, it is usually a reflection of them onto you, and should not be taken as fact. The idea was studied in depth by Sigmund Freud and is a "defence mechanism in which the individual attributes to other people impulses and traits that he himself has but cannot accept. It is especially likely to occur when the person lacks insight into his own impulses and traits."

That's an important point to take note of:

"Especially likely to occur when the person lacks insight into his own impulses and traits."

Again it's a case of, how can anybody, other than yourself, know what you're capable of, especially when they probably lack insight into themselves and their own ability? When somebody dismisses your chances, don't take it personally. Think about what they've said with the knowledge that you are the ultimate judge on what you can and will do. Again, as long as you are being honest with yourself and are willing to put the work in, I'd trust your own instincts over critics. Hey, critics and experts have always made mistakes. As long as you know that and understand that people are very good at projecting their own fears and failures on to you. As well as particularly, their own lack of ambition, you're on track!

"Our doubts are traitors,
And make us lose the good we oft might win,
By fearing to attempt."
William Shakespeare

Determining what's possible and impossible for you is the key!

In 1970, political thinker Zbigniew Brzezinski, wrote about our thoughts too. He points out that in the future, we won't even have to reason for ourselves, or that we won't know how to because the media will do it for us. The media will give us our definition of what's right and what's wrong (i.e. what is possible and impossible) and not only that, the moral choices and our (opposing) arguments. We will then regurgitate that, as our own point of view.

Of course, he was right, and of course, when is the media or anything "out in the world" going to give **you** the full picture about anything. I put it to you that, you're going to have to determine for yourself what is possible and impossible for you and then decide. You should look for your own truth and uniquely have a point of view on it. As with your goals and ambitions from the mundane to the profound, if it's important enough to have an opinion on, then it's important enough to have all the facts and think about it for yourself and decide what YOU think. Especially if it's something that you're going to base your life on. A decision taken in your youth might have an effect on the rest of your life and your level of happiness. You want to make the right ones as best as you can, because you wouldn't want to regret something as big as that. The good news though, is that there is always hope, in the words of Jesse Jackson, "Keep hope alive!"

You can only act to your fullest potential with all of the facts (or as much as you can get). It's always good to know what the bottom line is, as you have the ability to trust your own instincts and to know what is right or wrong for you, (looks good or not). Personally I'd rather have my own opinions than somebody else's forced on to me. I think that the word "forced" , although a strong word is appropriate and accurate in this case. Why would you dream of letting somebody else tell you what to think or do anyway? As the adage goes; *"Accept nothing as true that is not self evident",* and I would add *"to me",* not self evident to somebody else. Why? Because the whole world *can* be wrong!

The world is flat, believe me, I'm an expert!

If you lived in the 7th century BC, then *"SKY NEWS 7th Century BC edition"* and *"School Teacher Mrs Maurice"* as well as your *"Best friend McCarthy", "Pastor Friar", "Fox News panel expert"* (wooden 2×4 panel in those days) would be telling YOU that the earth was flat, and they'd swear on their eternal souls that it was! Unfortunately, they didn't have the luxury of disagreeing publicly in those days (unless they wanted to have the luxury of being barbecued at the stake!)

Question (Mother):

"Would you jump off a cliff if everybody else was doing it?"

Answer (boy):

"Yes, mother, I would, because you'd be first in the queue taking me over with you".

...the young boy might have a point! Just because you think that you can't dance or can't sing or can't do anything and the experts all agree, doesn't necessarily make it so! In fact most people are followers and will not take a stand for what they believe in for their own good, so how can they know what's right for you, when they in turn take their definition of what's possible and impossible for them from somebody else?

"It is not worth an intelligent man's time to be in the majority. By definition, there are already enough people to do that"
G. H. Hardy

The experts get it wrong: Big time!

Famous Misconceptions may be easy to ridicule now, but it's interesting to note that some of the most foolish statements of all time were given as basic facts and YOU would have been put in the "Looney bin" for stating otherwise. Now if some of the biggest conceptions and ideas in history can be wrong, could it be possible that your "smaller" negative ideas and conceptions about yourself and your actual potential might possibly be incorrect too? Let's take a closer look at a few examples…

The earth is flat…

It's a famous misconception that the people of the middle ages believed that the earth was flat….in actual fact, they didn't! It was determined a thousand years earlier, in the 6th Century BC, by Pythagoras the famous philosopher and mathematician, who advocated that the earth was a spherical shape. Even so, there was a point in time when people did indeed believe with all their hearts, that the earth was flat. Ptolemy, known as one of the greatest minds ever advocated that the earth was the centre of the universe and that the sun revolved around the earth! We can look back and laugh, but it's important to note that these were views advocated by the experts, scientists and the greatest minds of the day. It is all too easy to make "scientific" and value-judgments based upon what we take for granted today, and on subjective ever changing social norms, rather than look at the facts and decide on evidence, (or reality!) rather than bias and personal preconceptions….usually misconceptions. Even the greatest of minds make mistakes and evidently big ones, but that's part of human nature. You can't always trust the expert! The real issue lies in challenging misconceptions, and our negative preconceptions of ourselves. It has been said:

"Many people have difficulty letting go of misconceptions because the false concepts may be deeply ingrained in the mental map of an individual. Some people also don't like to be proven wrong and will continue clinging to a misconception in the face of evidence to the contrary. This is a known psychological phenomenon and is due to the lack of will or inability to re-evaluate information in a more objective way."

We're now talking about the root of the problem: intellectual integrity. You want to succeed in any field or achieve any goal in life then you need to be intellectually honest, to move to your highest potential! But we'll come back to that…some more classic expert advice and predictions:

"You better get secretarial work or get married."
Emmeline Snively, director of the Blue Book Book Modelling Agency, advising would-be model Marilyn Monroe in 1944.

"I would say that this does not belong to the art which I am in the habit of considering music."
A Oulibicheff, reviewing Beethoven's Fifth Symphony.

"Who the hell wants to hear actors talk?"
H. M. Warner, co-founder of Warner Brothers. (1927).

"The horse is here to stay but the automobile is only a novelty - a fad."
The president of the Michigan Savings Bank advising Henry Ford's lawyer not to invest in the Ford Motor Co. 1903.

"We don't like their sound, and guitar music is on the way out."
Decca Records, when they rejected The Beatles, 1962.

"Television won't last because people will soon get tired of staring at a plywood box every night."
Darryl Zanuck, movie producer, 20th Century Fox, 1946.

"... good enough for our transatlantic friends ... but unworthy of the attention of practical or scientific men."
British Parliamentary Committee, referring to Edison's light bulb, 1878.

"Sure-fire rubbish."
Lawrence Gilman, reviewing Porgy and Bess by George Gershwin in the New York Herald Tribune, 1935.

"If excessive smoking actually plays a role in the production of lung cancer, it seems to be a minor one."
W.C. Heuper, National Cancer Institute, 1954.

"The singer (Mick Jagger) will have to go; the BBC won't like him."
First Rolling Stones manager Eric Easton to his partner after watching them perform.

And finally, one of my favourites:

"It will be gone by June."
Variety, passing judgement on rock 'n roll in 1955.

…And all totally wrong!

Now, the good news is that all of these comments and opinions of the so called "experts", at the time, had absolutely no bearing on reality, the success of the product or the person. Imagine if they would have packed in and given up after listening to their foolish advice….no Beethoven, no Gershwin, no light bulb, no Beatles, no Mick Jagger, no television, no Monroe, no cars….imagine the face of the world today. All of these individuals had an additional piece of the puzzle, they could see the larger picture and could think "outside the box", they just continued on their course…and it really is that simple…they just did it! They put the work in and succeeded in changing history and the world we live in for ever. Doubt can be extremely destructive, William Shakespeare, wrote "Our doubts are traitors, and make us lose the good we oft might win, by fearing to attempt." He along with Monroe, Jagger and the others knew that doubt is over rated!

Taking a closer look….Lessons learned?

If we take a closer look at all of the comments, we notice a couple of important things. For one, they were incorrect predictions or misconceptions or just a foolish comment said at the time, but the most important key point is that they had no bearing on reality or the outcome. Why? Because belief, perspective, proving things, opinions, and points of view are all variable, human and imperfect and ever changing…The truth is the truth, it just is. Statements, belief, declarations or opinions on the matter have no bearing on the fact, either way. The problem, lays with the person's statements, not with ability to succeed or fail, it is only an opinion. Is it valid, is it true? Taking a look at our previous examples, it is curious to note that the various statements, beliefs, declarations or opinions had no bearing on the outcome. Why? Because there is always a bottom line based on fact, which stands alone, separate to us or our thoughts and opinions. Now the previous naysayers could have believed and said whatever they wanted to about failure and success, it had no bearing on the truth: that's why "belief" is indeed NOT absolute, and "Truth" is. It is separate to us, it doesn't need our participation or agreement of you or the experts….belief does, and that's the flaw and that's why the experts get it wrong and thats why we shouldn't always trust our own temporary emotions or thoughts on a matter. Emotions change, as do feelings. We feel optimistic and happy one day and the next, we feel sad and upset. That's fine, as long as we remember that our points of view, opinions, belief, perspective change with our emotions and cannot really be taken as fact or as a true indication of what is to be. It's "Belief", what people usually want, and it has nothing to do with truth…as you can believe anything you want to, regardless of the fact of the matter and can be based on false negative opinions as well as social norms that might not even be true as well!

Doubt and Opinions are over rated!

"Belief" can be a barrier to success and achievement! We should strive to "know". Knowing and knowledge, doesn't involve opinion or even belief, as our opinion or belief has no affect on truth or the light. Belief is a barrier.

Truth IS!

Why you should dance, if that's what you feel you want to do!

If you've always dreamed of dancing then you should go ahead and start your journey. The fact of the matter is that if you take any kind of positive step, you will advance to your own truth and bring it into a successful reality and fact, regardless of what you feel or may have felt before you took any kind of action. Now, the question is, what is truth?

Truth just is what it is…"Your truth" and "my truth" is not. Truth is not subjective or affected by foolish predictions or the smart comments of the so called experts. When I say "Truth is", I mean that that is your *actual* chances of success in a matter where you **take simple logical steps to your required destination**. If you take logical small simple steps, incrementally, then, if you stick to the right plan, then you will arrive at your required destination no matter what, regardless of fear, thoughts, opinions etc. Remember, a lot of people make comments and ask questions not to "know", but to "believe". Believing something which is easy to accept, doesn't challenge them or affect their daily life too much. People will believe what they want and *not what they don't want to* *believe*. People ask questions to hear a response that they want to hear, or fits into a defined space that they have created, usually if the truth doesn't fit, into their understanding or belief system (*for example*) then it is disregarded, ignored etc. Even so, it's irrelevant because **a person's opinion has nothing to do with your chances of success or achievement** and the truth or the fact of the matter. An opinion is just a thought, it actively does nothing unless you allow it to change your behaviour. Your behaviour can affect achievement, but thoughts and opinion have no real affect on reality. An example…

I have a magic time machine and a magic space ship! I travel back in time to 7th Century BC and take a nice spin around the earth…great!

Every person on earth is certain, they believe, they "know", they are of the opinion……the laws of nature and experts as well as the greatest minds on earth, the experts, all have a default position….the earth is flat and the earth is at the centre of the universe!

(And we might as well add that you can fall off the edge of it too, if you travel too far west!)

Of course they are completely wrong. Totally! Because they do not KNOW they only thought they did…..and thoughts change nothing in reality.

Me inside my magic machine, orbiting the earth…..I have true knowledge…I KNOW…..I do not have to believe, or have an opinion about it….I KNOW, crazy nutters on earth BELIEVE…

Would it be a wise decision to base your life on information that is incorrect and false? To build your life on other people's, as well as your own misconceptions and incorrect opinions. No…of course not and this is the most important key point to consider! Every successful plan needs honest information and you can't get very far, or reach your true potential and destination without honest information as opposed to opinion or belief, no matter how convinced they or you think you are. True Success: Intellectual integrity. Organisation. Planning and then implementing your plan precisely. Your opinions on your ability might be wrong… that's a good thing…because we never know how far we can go…there are no restrictions, except the restrictions we place on ourselves. If I put one foot in front of the other and walk, then logically, I will move forward, regardless of my changing thoughts, belief or opinion on the matter. If I do it, and go through the motions, the outcome is assured. I will move forward. If we let our emotion and thoughts dictate our action then we'd probably be stuck on the same spot, worrying about the consequences of taking a simple step, rather than just doing it! If I believe that my feet will be swallowed up by the earth, then that too is just as crazy as many of the silly excuses and restrictions that we place on ourselves daily e.g. what will my friends think? I've never done anything like that before, I don't think I have what it takes, I'll never be able to dance etc…Remember the outcome is assured, do not fear! Life is scientific in that sense, take a small step, and then take another. One step plus one step is two steps forward! Once you're moving forward, your own doubts and the foolish expert advice of your peers will be relegated to the past and you can turn back and wave, fortunately knowing that you didn't base your decision to act on a negative opinion of your own making, or from others for that matter!

Why is it necessary to have accurate information though? Well, let's say that you've decided to disregard your feelings and fear, and started to move forward in your chosen field, with small steps. You are moving forward, in the right direction. It's important that you don't forget that a) things change b) you are human, and your doubts, fear and negative feelings will sometimes overcome your ability to continue on that course and c) the course is not necessarily a linear one. An example…let's say that I really want to go to the park. It's my lifelong ambition to play on the swings and run around in the green fields! The park itself is only a few blocks away but I have never looked at a map to see, I have never been to the park before and I've heard from others (who also have never been to the park) that it's really hard to get to. I've heard lot's of rumours about the park's location and different opinions on whether it exists at all! Nevertheless, I have a feeling it exists and I want to do it! The wisest thing to do would be to firstly, understand what a "park" is. Yes, that sounds crazy! But, you need to know what it looks like so you don't miss it. Good. Secondly, determine it's location in relation to your current location. Then research things like distance, obstacles and other relevant information on the journey. Thirdly, make a plan, prepare and start moving toward the park. If you come up to an obstacle then continue through it, round it or over it, until eventually, you'll be relaxing in the park in no time!

Pretty simple really! Oh no….not for us….we must complicate the situation! Imagine if instead of understanding what I'd have to do to get to the park and making and implementing a plan of action to get there, I'd stood in the same spot, stationary, staring at my toes! Imagine that I didn't bother to find out what a park was and had listened to other peoples' opinions and myths about the park, who, in turn had never even been to the park or even understood what it was. Imagine if I would not have had the courage to make one simple step toward the park due to misplaced fear and opinion. "Imagine" is exactly the right word…it would remain a fantasy in my mind. If I would have based my actions on logic then I'd be at my destination.

On the other hand, if we base our actions or non action on beliefs and thoughts, we are setting ourselves up for failure from the outset. The key is to remember that logical planned action will always prevail. What have you got to lose? It takes up more energy to worry about the consequences of a given action then actually carrying it out and following it through, most of the time! The question is, Why? Why do we allow doubts and fears to dictate our action or lack of it, when in actual fact, doubs and fears are usually illogical and blown out of proportion in our own minds. It's just so much easier to do something then to worry about the consequences. Before we take a look at that, let's not forget one more thing. Direction is key! I could be extremely enthusiastic, moving forward one step at a time…but walking in the opposite direction! With any ambition or dream, it's important to count the cost involved in advancing, without prejudice. That way you have a higher chance of arriving at your destination speedily. It's important to count the cost, and to do your reconnaissance *in advance*, so you understand your mission, potential obstacles, have a plan for them, and know what direction you're going and most importantly, understand WHAT you are doing and WHY? That way, logic alone will tell you that your odds are not only increased of success, but the journey will be a lot more enjoyable, as you might be prepared for any set backs or the unexpected along the way. Remember, no fear. An honest way to success is simple thought, planning, and putting your foot in front of the other. What have you got to lose by taking small steps at a time to achieve any of your goals, no matter what that may be, dance or otherwise?

Could it be that achieving your goals is as simple as that? Just a case of "doing it"? I would say "yes". Sometimes the most profound truths are quite simple, but it is we ourselves who complicate the situation, we want a complicated quick fix, as opposed to hearing that there is no easy way to get from A to Z with one jump. It might take time and mental strength, but if you are willing to focus on your goals, are willing to be intellectually honest from the outset, make a logical plan and just take one step at a time, then reality will increasingly start to look like your dreams coming true. The important point is that you can't cheat; you have to go through the motions. You'll have to work hard and you'll have to be mentally strong and focused. If you can do those things, then you will understand the secret of success.

Can we learn from the attitude of our Children?

"The only thing that interferes with my learning is my education"
Albert Einstein

I think we could learn a lot about ourselves by looking at the behaviour and attitude of our children. The things that we all used to be! It's amazing how the magic qualities are literally bred out of us. Children are full of hope and are dreamers! My opinion is pretty simple: we need to shut up and listen to our children and we might actually get somewhere and start enjoying life. Sir Ken Robinson, former board member of the National Ballet recently delivered a speech on Creativity and how the "education" system fails us when it comes to creativity. This is obviously clear to see! I get so many emails and talk to so many adults, mature grown up people, saying that "they always wanted to dance", "always wanted to do this" etc…but my parents made me do this or that and now I'm a city banker, accountant or whatever, namely doing stuff that I don't like…They wish they would have done this earlier…

Why didn't you do what you wanted to do? Let's take a look:

- My parents didn't let me
- I didn't believe I could
- I wasn't trained
- I come from an academic family
- People thought that it was silly
- I didn't have the courage to follow my heart

Oscar Wilde said "Most people are other people. Their thoughts are somebody else's opinions". I agree. I personally discovered this at a very young age. Unfortunately some people never do and will live their lives never to do what they really wanted to do, always waiting for somebody to lead them to the light. I have some news: they aren't coming! We shouldn't forget that, as adults we are trained to censor and subdue ourselves, to wear social masks and to hide our emotions. Let's be frank, the only time you really get the truth out of an adult is when they are drunk!
Young children on the other hand don't know about these social rules. They are spontaneous, they will run riot and free! Take a child to a park and he or she will run and play and dance and be happy to just express themselves in the mud and sand, and they don't care who is watching or what other people think. A child will show there feelings in an honest way. Now, as adults, this kind

of honest behaviour has been indoctrinated out of us, so that a grown mature adult doesn't have the courage to do something that they really want to do, due to other people, that they do not even know, and their opinions. Not only do some people not have the ability but also don't even know how!

There are consequences for this kind of suppression. The basic survival mechanisms that a child has are foolishly bred out of us all...the same survival mechanisms that we all need as adults too. For example, if a child doesn't like you, they will show it! They won't take the time to cover it up and lie to your face. They sense people's deceitfulness and evil and have no problem in showing it! Most people have experienced the relative or friend that is a complete idiot and obviously a viper, who is invited around the house. As a child, you can sense it a million miles off, but can't understand why your family puts up with it and force you to pretend that you are pleased to see them too! It's this honesty and judgement that we need later, all the more in the real world, to protect us from the manipulators, thieves and just plain foolish people who we all have to put up with at points during our lives.

Can we change all this? One thing which intrigues me is how you feel as you get older? What have you learned? What would you do

if you could start again? I think it would be pretty cool to work out the answer BEFORE you get old, that would be great!
I recently spent a day in Birmingham teaching a dance workshop for school children and it was so refreshing! We sang "Willy Wonka" songs and it was so fun! Ha Ha! Then on the way back on the train I sat near six naughty children causing mischief…. Ha Ha…they were so funny! I think that I was the only one laughing at their jokes! And finally yesterday I met a wonderful child called "Jacob" who really made my day and tried to steal a girl that I liked….and he succeeded and he was only eight! Ha Haaaaa! Childish? Not at all! Well, I always tell my best friends "let's go to a playground and play!" they think I'm nuts! I have a lovely friend who lives in Slovenia and she has a playground in front of her house - when we got in after midnight one night we spent the best time, playing in the playground.

Childish, crazy, a waste of time? No, I'll tell you what's crazy:

On my way to catch my train to Birmingham from Euston I was in a packed line on the underground walking to get the train. I can honestly say that I felt like a beast being herded to the slaughter house! It's been a while since I've been in the morning rush hour and I had to turn around and take it in and laugh out loud! Is this what it's all about? Go to school, to get trained so that I can join the cue of expressionless droids at Euston or London Bridge on my way to a job that I hate to make money for somebody that I don't know, go on holiday for two weeks, go partying on Friday night and start again on Monday, so that I can pay the bills and do it all again and again first thing every Monday morning. No thank you! I'll go play in the playground and sing "Willy Wonka" songs!

In my experience I have learned something….your teachers, your parents and people in authority over you are generally not the foremost experts and authority on anything! They repeat what has been told to them: repeat, repeat, repeat! Generally, they do not think for themselves at all. They will impose their failures and beliefs on you! They'll advise YOU to go and work as a slave as an accountant, doctor, lawyer, shop assistant, street cleaner, carpenter or plumber. PLUS tell you that that is "good" and that is a success. Why? Because that's all they know! Nobody has told them that they can do whatever they want to. Now if that's what YOU enjoy then that is a good thing, but if you do it to satisfy your parents or because that's what everyone else thinks you should do (then you will have to live with it and you are off your rocker!)

Now, of course, not all adults are full of it…just most. It doesn't take a rocket scientist to work it out…just take a look at the world around us, open a newspaper, turn on the news….what happened! Look at the way we treat our children! Look at the murders, wars and hate….I say that we should put an 8 year old in charge of every country and we'd have a fairer, happier world for sure! (and something else sticks in my mind regarding children; the way in which we treat them and often bring them up to turn out as madcap as us!)

I know somebody, very close to me, who was physically and mentally abused. I've known this person for a long time and have seen the bruises. This person's family loved to beat them, not smack, beat. It has affected them forever. They beat with belts, metal spoons, bamboo sticks, smashed spatulas on them; they even possessed a whip! How on earth can you ever abuse a child and be sane! It is clear that these people were just following their own vicious desires and were probably abused themselves… the point is that these people believed that what they were doing was right. They truly believed that they were doing good. I mean, look at what our leaders are doing around the world, look at the homeless on the street. Adults do not have a clue and are so stubborn that they will never compromise and think logically or even in a logical way. They will encourage you to be like everybody else and NOT follow your dreams, and they will do it with a smile believing that they are right. People die every day for their religions and they kill everyday for their beliefs. It's our adults that do this! Our mature grown ups! We should all take a look at our children and the way in which they think and behave. Wouldn't it be interesting if we were all childlike (not childish) and expressed ourselves the way we want. Real freedom. Mentally and physically, as opposed to repression and unfulfilled dreams of most adults. No, no, not for me and it doesn't have to be that way for you!

How to feel great…Have some fun!

OK, time for some child's play regarding the easiest way to feel great and stay in shape! It's really easy to change your outlook and feel great, and I'm going to let you into the secret! How to stay in shape, how to stay energised, how to just be well! Now, before I let you into the secret…I have to admit that I stole it, from probably the greatest actor ever: Marlon Brando. It's the secret weapon that I pull out when I'm feeling down or overworked.

As a choreographer and dance teacher, it's also my job to give advice on *how much* to dance and practice and exercise tips and all of that. But again, do you want to hear something that costs nothing and is so simple, that doesn't involve a 15 step plan and your hard earned cash, only a little determination? I always tell my students that the best way to stay healthy and keep fit is a) to dance and b) to run (although that's not the secret!). Trust me, I have heard every excuse conceivable in the book, why this is not possible. It's quite entertaining to hear the same excuses from so many different people! It's quite simple; although you might have to wake up 45 minutes earlier in the morning. All you have to do is invest in a good quality pair of trainers (sneakers) and run daily.... That's it! But of course, they would rather quote scientific theories on shock impact as if they're experts in Chondromalacia, Chronic exertional compartment syndrome, Great excuse syndrome as well as other knee disorders...Anything not to, in the words of Nike "Just do it!" (...Interestingly, the same people who take such an interest in the sciences are not too worried at the inhaling of toxins and drinking poison in the pub every night!)

Anyway, I digress!

It's really simple and is also the perfect way to jump into dance and any physical activity, especially for absolute beginners. Although it is very simple, it's something that so many people are unable to do. The number one way to lose weight and get into dance and get your backside moving! The bad news is that you won't want to hear it. It's probably too simple for you to accept!

The Secret

Marlon Brando. The man. Marlon Brando had the most amazing ability to lose weight. I mean, seriously, he would go from being a very healthy lean looking movie star to a massively overweight man, and then back again, in very short periods of time....But how!?? He was once asked in an interview, "How do you lose weight so quickly?" Now, you'd be surprised at his answer. Did it involve an army of Hollywood trainers? No! Did it involve subscribing to nonsensical unhealthy scam diets? No! It was completely free...and very easy to do. He would close the curtains, close the doors, put on a great piece of music full blast... and just go crazy! Yes, just move to the music. No choreography, no nothing! He said that he just copied the Hula dancers that he watched, with all that movement. You are a human being, with natural rhythm....Why do you need to learn to go enjoy a great happy song? You don't. And I mean, go crazy...Just do whatever you feel like, manoeuvre like a crazy beast...Just lose control for once. Feel free to lose your inhibitions and be free! Hey, nobody's watching, so who gives a damn anyway!

Marlon Brando filmed and vacationed in Hawaii, and was inspired and impressed by the natural movements e.g. Natural dance like the Samburu tribe dance, in Africa. Forget this nonsense that you have to "learn" how to do this, or "learn" how to do that or that you can only lose weight and keep fit and "feel good" with a yearly membership at the top gym, that you hardly attend anyway, repeating mechanical, totally non natural, robotic movements in front of a flashing box. Which is a totally new phenomenon anyway. You tell me where the healthiest people in the world are. Not in the same locations as the countries with the most gyms, I bet!

As every Philosopher has said, it's always a case of "unlearning" rather than "learning". And one more thing, mentally, you will feel great afterwards too. For once, really do something spontaneous and give it a try! That is my personal feel good keep fit advice: the technique that I employ when I'm feeling down! Now, as always, it

might be too complicated for you to do something so simple - but why not give it a try! It's the perfect place to start for a beginner and I guarantee that you'll feel great afterwards and really be in a better position to advance and learn, as well as keep in shape.
My Top 5 personally recommended songs!

1) "Wanna be startin something" by Michael Jackson
2) "Venus" by Bananarama
3) "I will survive" by Gloria Gaynor
4) "Manic Monday" by the Bangles
5) "Puttin on the Ritz" performed by Fred Astaire

And any Michael Jackson track....Good luck! Think about your mental ability to try new things and not disregard something that may indeed help you. That simple thing might be something that you could use to progress. Don't disregard anything just because it sounds too simple. Advancement in the physical really does start in your head.

Autobiography in Five Short Chapters by Portia Nelson

From, *there's a Hole in My Sidewalk*,

I:

I walk down the street.
There is a deep hole in the sidewalk.
I fall in.
I am lost…
I am helpless.
It is not my fault.
It takes forever to find my way out.

II:

I walk down the same street.
There is a deep hole in the sidewalk.
I pretend I don't see it.
I fall in.
I can't believe I am in the same place.
But it isn't my fault.
It still takes a long time to get out.

III:

I walk down the same street.
There is a deep hole in the sidewalk.
I see it there.
I still fall in…It's a habit.
My eyes are open.
I know where I am.
It is my fault.
I get out immediately.

IV:

I walk down the same street.
There is a deep hole in the sidewalk.
I walk around it.
I walk down another street.

I first read this poem in Sean Covey's book "the 7 Habits of Highly effective teens". I highly recommend it for anybody wanting to affect positive change in their life. His father wrote a book called "the 7 habits of highly effective people", which is great also, but the principles are exactly the same in the "younger" version, but it's so much easier to read and has really great pictures! I find that good news is usually simple and doesn't have to be complicated. Just like this poem. You'd be surprised at what you can achieve if you just make the most obvious changes and decide to become proactive and start to make positive decisions. I think that this poem sums it up well. If you're fed up of not being able to dance or not being able to do something that you really want to do, then it doesn't make sense to complain or even accept the results because they are completely logical and expected results of your *current actions*. If you want different results then you will have to make a decision to do something different. The actual act of doing something "different", is not the hard part, but making that conscious decision is what challenges people the most. Have you ever thought, why don't we keep our New Year resolutions? Every year we promise to lose weight, or do this or do that, but for most it usually turns into nothing. Why? Well, I would put it to you that it's because you don't want change bad enough. Because when you do, then that will be that and you will start doing what you want and achieving your goals.

Put yourself in a situation where you have no choice but to succeed, where failure is not an option.

Napoleon Hill told the story of a warrior who lived a long time ago; he had to go and fight a battle and had to make a decision that would ensure victory. He had to go and attack a massive mighty army, and his small force was greatly outnumbered. He packed the ships with supplies and loaded the soldiers onboard and set sail to attack. After he arrived on the shores and unpacked his equipment and men, he gave the order to set fire to the ships! Before the battle he made an impassioned speech and said, "You see the boats going up in smoke. That means that we cannot leave these shores alive unless we win! *We win – or we perish*!", and they did indeed win; they had no choice or other course of action! If you want to start achieving your goals, once and for all, then you need to get that kind of burning desire, where you make a conscious decision to dance, succeed or whatever…without the fear of failure, because you cannot accept the alternative.

The "Great Chicago Fire" in 1871, burned down several square miles of down town Chicago and was one of the biggest fires of the 19th century. The morning after the fire, the shop owners and merchants went to have a look at the smouldering remains of what used to be their factories and stores. They all met together and had a conference to decide what they should do. Should they attempt to salvage what they could from the ruins and rebuild? Or leave town and start over at a more promising part of the country. Well in the end they all concluded that they should cut their losses and leave Chicago, all except one. The one that remained stood up and pointed at what used to be his store and said, "Gentlemen, on that very spot I will build the world's greatest store, no matter how many times it may burn down". And of course Marshal Field kept his word and his department store went on to become iconic. He had that fire inside him and there was no alternative in his mind, failure was not even an option.

Sometimes people get so sick and tired of failure or of not being able to do something and see everyone else around them doing it…that it can drive them down the path to success. This process sometimes takes a long time. It might take years and years for some to realise that they can't handle not implementing change and start taking some action, because they just can't stand the alternative any longer. This is a pity, because if they can come to that realisation in later life, then they can do it earlier and enjoy the benefits for longer. The bottom line is that it's just a mental decision. If you want it then go and get it. Or at the very least open your mouth and ask for it. You must at least try, what have you got to lose anyway?

I want to tell you a story about a dear friend of mine who was "sick and tired of being sick and tired", about one of his lifelong dreams. Before I do that, I just want you to take a look at a poem by Jessie B. Rittenhouse called "My wage", and have a good think about it. She sums it up really well, that universal truth, that the difference between you achieving a goal and not, is actually pretty small. Napoleon Hill put it this way, and makes the same point, "no more effort is required to aim high in life, to demand abundance and prosperity, than is required to accept misery and poverty". The key is to realise that at an early age, so you can enjoy the benefits **now**, instead of living in regret later, when you can't do anything about it. There is always hope and you can change today!

"My wage" by Jessie B. Rittenhouse

"I bargained with Life for a penny,
And Life would pay no more,
however I begged at evening
when I counted my scanty store.

For Life is a just employer,
He gives you what you ask,
but once you have set the wages,
why, you must bear the task.

I worked for a menial's hire,
only to learn, dismayed,
that any wage I had asked of Life,
Life would have willingly paid."

Yes, the secret is that whatever you ask for is what you get. The key is to speak up, loud and clear, while you can still enjoy the benefits. Just like Simon Dover did!

Simon's story

Simon Dover, a successful business man, owner of one of the top chains of bakeries in London, which he built up from scratch, was fed up! Although he was a successful businessman who, on the surface looked liked he had everything, there was just one thing that always bugged him. He was afraid of dancing and felt that he couldn't dance. This had a major impact on the quality of his social interactions and he hadn't danced for years. Whenever he went to weddings or had the guts to go into a club, he would just stand at the side and have a drink, because there was no way on earth that he could go anywhere near the dance floor or even a few steps away from the bar. That would be impossible! The problem for Simon is that this had gone on for years and years and now he was fed up! He couldn't take it anymore and it got to the point where the unhappiness out weighed the fear of enquiring what he could do about it. Although, in his mind, it was impossible for him to dance or be taught, he plucked up the courage to go to the dance schools website and make contact. This was really embarrassing for him and a big step, but that was no worse than the years and years of embarrassment and the empty feeling at the end of any night out.

Hey, he thought there was no hope, so what did he have to lose anyway?

I asked him to tell me what he wanted me to do for him and what he wanted to get out of this, what were his aims? The bottom line was that there was no hope for him and that he thought that he would just give it a crack and attempt to learn a few steps, for the fun of it and there was a big wedding abroad coming up, that he had to go to, and it would be nice not to go straight to the bar when the music started. He went on to say that he was kind of large and shy as well. Interesting, I thought. The great thing is that he was totally honest and up front from the beginning. He had nothing to lose and everything to gain. No ego and no expectations…he could literally, not get any worse…so it was all good! We arranged to meet at the dance studios. Simon later went on to describe the fear that he felt when he entered the building and how it literally hit him with force and how it made him feel quite intimidated. Well as I saw him across the canteen above the studio, I thought to myself, "this guy looks great and very established". He explained how he felt and I told him not to worry at all. After we got started, I asked him to show me how he usually dances. He told me that he doesn't at all, and hasn't ever.

"Interesting", I thought, but of course that's never a problem!

The curious thing is that because he had nothing to lose and everything to gain, he just listened and repeated and repeated (and repeated!) until he started to get it! After a few private lessons he said that he now had the courage to try and come to a public dance class. He came prepared, early and ready to go. He hid in the corner and tried his hardest, but at the end of the day, he survived and met lots of like-minded people. It's a different world on the other side of the glass and everyone is in the same boat trying to learn. Now Simon started to come more and more regularly; within two to three months he had moved himself up to the front of the class and people were asking him how long he had come for. Simon thought that this was unbelievable! He was just a baker who couldn't dance at all! But the fact of the matter is that he was progressing because he took action and the first "impossible step". But that's not the end of the story.

Simon came out for a drink with some friends, one of which was a casting director who was looking for one more male who could act, for a commercial. He said that Simon looked perfect for the job and could he come along to the casting? Now you have to remember that this is all a big joke to Simon…a MD of a big company, being asked to be in commercials…this was all too surreal! Well, within a few weeks Simon was on television in a music commercial! After that, he was contacted by one of the biggest Dairy companies in the world who thought that he would make a perfect Baker in their commercial too…big money and worldwide!

Simon's life had transformed in a matter of a few weeks and his confidence had increased to an unbelievable extent. He had learned to let go of his fear and to just relax. He had learned to dance and he had made lots of new friends along the way and now was on his way to becoming a star too! Wow! The transformation from that first email to now is shocking! But the most important thing in Simon's story is that he took the first fearful step and then he just proceeded to take more little steps. Just small steps, nothing immediately life changing or earth shattering and look at the positive transformation, unbelievable. Well actually quite believable. He had been so fed up that he felt that the alternative to all this was just not worth it. He was fed up with that and would have it no longer. It's interesting if you think about it. He is exactly the same person that wrote that first email, just with a different attitude and perspective. He has taken the steps, gained the experience and understood that it was just fear, but that it was unfounded. He survived in the end, had lots of fun and most importantly came to realise that he was absolutely incorrect to say that things were "impossible" for him to do. He was wrong, it was very possible and he did it. It would be a real tragedy if he didn't pluck up the courage to just take that step and write the email. Maybe he might have written it 10 years later. That would have been 10 years lost. Don't lose another day! Trust me, you don't know what you can actually do and achieve, no matter what you may think…*nothing* is impossible. And even if your "goals" seem impossible, then, you should still go for them, because you'll have nothing to lose and miracles do happen! So that is that. Oh, and one more thing…the wedding!

Well, well…Simon travels off to the wedding and boy did he have a surprise lined up for his best friend! During the dancing the announcement came over the loud speakers to clear the dance floor…Simon was going to dance solo. He was going to perform! The music came on, he did it, the whole place erupted in applause and the deed was done! He had won, he had overcome another challenge that he thought was impossible and not only had he overcome it, he obliterated self doubt to pieces! Oh and one more thing, while he's at the wedding he meets a girl who thinks that he's amazing and is so impressed by his amazing dancing skills. She moves over to London and they're now getting married! Now that's a great story. Simon is an amazing man and I am honoured to be part of somebody's dreams coming true.

Take the small step. You have nothing to lose. What else would you do with your time? Can you spend it more wisely than working toward your honest goals, dreams and aspirations? Think about answering it now, because it is a question that you will ask one day, hopefully sooner rather than later. Take a look at the character of "Edmond Dantes" in Alexander Dumas' "The Count of Monte Cristo". For the first couple of years of his imprisonment in the Château d'If, he sat banging his head against the solid rock wall doing nothing but turning to madness and then after a long period of time he realised something. He started scratching at the wall, and small fragments would fall off, admittedly they were almost invisible, but after a few hours, he had scrapped off about a handful. He calculated that if he had done this for two years, instead of squandering his time, then he could have dug a passage "two feet across and twenty feet deep". And "realising this, the prisoner regretted not having devoted the long hours that had already passed, ever so slowly, to the task…however slow the work, how much would he have achieved in the six or so years that he had spent buried in this dungeon! The idea fired him with renewed enthusiasm". The message is clear: The time you spend pondering and toiling about doing something could just as easily be used to do it and probably complete the task! You're not going to travel backwards away from your goal so it is a lot wiser to just push ahead. Time can be an ally. Rather than staying stationary and regretting not moving forward, logic alone will tell you that with time you will eventually get to your destination no matter how slowly you progress and a lot quicker than not moving at all!

…Take hope from Edmond Dante (and Simon!). Edmond escaped the terrible dungeon of the Château d'If by slow, seemingly tedious fruitless digging through solid rock…but over time it worked for him and he achieved his goal. All you need is time and a small amount of action toward your desired goal and you'll be on the right track.

Part 2: Celebrity Fitness

You are what you eat

"Dieting is no substitute for exercise"

Dr Mileham Hayes

The foundation of a healthy lifestyle is diet and exercise. The two have a symbiotic relationship and both are keys to your well being. It's also important to realise that "diet is no substitute for exercise". You can eat a healthy balanced diet and still be unfit and perform well below your optimum without exercise, and you will perform well below your optimum level if you exercise regularly but have a poor unhealthy diet. You need to have both; a healthy balance and you will see amazing results in your fitness, lifestyle and general well being!

We process food at different rates, as we all have a unique metabolism. But it is quite clear that there is no magic formula or secret diet that will work for all…because we are all different, but it is possible to find a metabolic balance, where you nourish yourself to your optimum level whilst consuming the right healthy amounts of fats, which leads to a healthy balance, your well being and your ideal bodyweight. One thing is quite clear; healthy, logical moderation is key…quick fix diets and popular fads are temporary solutions that can damage your long term health and are not solid foundations for a healthy lifestyle. If you become aware of how you eat and the different reasons why, including any psychological attachments that you may have to certain foods, then you can become more in tune with your body and its needs and change your lifestyle and improve the quality of your life for the better.

Some basic advice

Let's face it, we're all pretty busy and don't have the time to be keeping a daily food diary and counting every calorie that we consume with every mouthful wherever we may be. And the good news is that it's just totally unnecessary! The bottom line is this: You want change or you don't. You want to live a healthy lifestyle and be the best energetic person you can be or you don't. If you really do, then the good news is that if you follow some simple logical guidelines then you will see a transformation over time naturally and other people will notice it too. It is pretty simple when you break it down. If you don't exercise and you eat too much, especially when you aren't hungry, you are wearing your body down and eating in excess. In today's modern culture with Hollywood dieting, energy bars, energy drinks, and quick snacks it is easy to forget our "normal" appetite and hunger levels. The healthy idea of eating when your hungry and stopping when you feel full have been smashed and replaced with, "I'll have a quick bite on the way to the office" or "I'll eat when I have time". If you focus on eating within a natural framework and only eat when you are hungry and stop when you are comfortably full, you will begin to retrain your mind and body and retain your natural body weight in a healthy sustained way. Crazy diets and quick fixes are not necessary!

A Simple Healthy framework

What is a healthy framework? Well, a healthy frame work is simply, **three healthy meals a day**. And if you are hungry**, two healthy snacks daily as well**. This is your foundation and a solid daily framework that will give you all that you need to function healthily and to your optimum level as well attain and maintain a healthy body weight. It generally makes sense to have a fairly substantial meal, as early as possible in the day to give you energy and to give you a kick start and keep you going with a healthy sustained energy release throughout the morning. But it is also important to remember that you eat, within the frame work, when you feel comfortable and it may not be feasible due to time restraints or other everyday factors, to have a very large breakfast first thing in the morning and would rather have a larger meal later in the day. This is absolutely fine, as it is your body and different strategies work for different types of people. You need to find out what works best for you and what makes you comfortable within the natural healthy framework.

Before we take a closer look at the various types of healthy macronutrients that the body needs to function healthily I should add one more important thing. Metabolic balance and a healthy food intake will help you focus naturally on the right foods for you and increase the level of your well being. After you have felt and observed the effect of positive dietary change you will not feel the urge to eat unhealthily and give up your energy and well being because of some temporary cravings that only give you short term pleasure and a quick high (and can leave you feeling dejected afterwards). They are usually physiological level issues, and will be addressed when you start to maintain a healthy balanced diet, naturally. Until that point it is important to keep sight of your goal and if you are over weight or unhappy with your lifestyle, to follow the most simple advice in the book. This might sound crazy, but if you follow this simple advice you will accelerate toward your goals: **Stop eating foods that you know make you fat, quick fix snacks that give you short term pleasure at the expense of your long term well being!**

Yes, it's that simple, and it's a decision for you to make, when you feel comfortable enough to do it. I guarantee you that, you cannot fail if you stick to a healthy balanced diet, but the choice is yours. You cannot fail if you simply eat the right foods for your body and overcome the urges, bad habits and food cravings that you know are detrimental to your mental and physical well being. Why not take a look at it from a different psychological level. If you had diabetes or heart disease, you would be advised by your doctor to stop eating certain foods, and the probability is that you would do it to preserve your life and well being so that you can enjoy all that it has to offer. I say that you, right now, have the chance to preserve your life and well being and really live life to the maximum by changing your outlook and diet and becoming a better version of who you are today. And that means that you may, want to take an honest look at your fat intake and those unhealthy foods that you *know* are detrimental to your health and cut them out. Just do it! Keep sight of your longer term goals and you'll be amazed at how it will get easier and easier, once you get going…the key, is to get going! Let's take a closer look at healthy eating and what the body needs, namely, Carbohydrates, proteins and fats.

Different types of Carbohydrates

There are two major types of Carbohydrates in foods: Simple and Complex. Simple carbohydrates (also known as "simple sugars") include glucose, lactose, sucrose, fructose and galactose, which are found in the sugar that we use in our tea, honey, some fruits as well as in milk and dairy products. Obviously, fruit and milk products are a lot better to consume compared to pure sugar and sweets because they contain other important nutrients like calcium, fibre and other vitamins. As opposed to pure refined sugar, in fizzy drinks for example, which might give you a quick short term burst of energy (and no other nutrients), but will go straight to your cells to be stored…and not invisibly or without consequences I hasten to add! Complex carbohydrates on the other hand are starches and contain nutrients, complicated sugars as well as fibre. Complex carbohydrates serve as a much more efficient and healthy fuel for the body and the nutrients and fibre, when broken down by the body, are stored and can easily be converted into energy, for when it is needed, in a slow release efficient way.

Another type of carbohydrate, found in foods which have lost their goodness, vitamins and minerals, due to refinement, are called "refined complex carbohydrates". They have had there skins and fibres removed and consequently, behave in the same way as simple carbohydrates, causing insulin production to increase and can be found in white flour, white rice and other "refined" foods that have lost that natural goodness. Additionally, white bread and other refined carbohydrates are usually combined with hydrogenated fats and pure sugar to improve the taste…not so good!

Complex Carbohydrates

Include: Whole grains, whole wheat pasta (i.e. Brown), brown bread, brown rice, Muesli, Potatoes, Cauliflower, Tomatoes, Onions, Kidney beans, Carrots, Cabbage, lentils, broccoli.

Simple Carbohydrates

Include: White bread, sugar, white pasta, cakes, fizzy drinks, fruit juices, chocolate, jams, most processed cereals, alcoholic drinks and all products made with white flour.

Consumption of these types of carbohydrate causes your blood sugar level to rise at drastically different rates. And it is important that your blood sugar level is regulated, guarding against heart disease and diabetes, for example. When you consume simple carbohydrates, it effectively raises your hormone insulin stimulation very quickly, whose job it is to regulate and keep the sugar level at a normal healthy level. This is because simple carbohydrates are absorbed very quickly into the blood stream, quickly raising the blood sugar level. Complex (unrefined) carbohydrates, on the other hand release sugar into the blood stream at a sustained slow rate over a much longer period. They are also rich in fibre. The key, is sustained healthy consumption and the release of its goodness over time as opposed to a quick fix, that doesn't last and is detrimental to your health.

Fibre

Fibre is found in unrefined grains and complex carbohydrates. It helps your digestive system work well, which is integral to your feeling of well being and fibre naturally fills you up. Consequently, you are unlikely to over eat as you will naturally feel full when your body has had the right amount of goodness. You might notice that a bowl of porridge (complex carbohydrate) fills you up, but a bowl of cornflakes (simple carbohydrate) for example, might not, even though they have the same amount of calories… so don't be fooled into thinking that less calories equals more healthy! Balance is the key. It's important to have a lot of fibre in your diet as it guards against obesity, bowel cancer and diabetes. The goodness is found in nuts, fruits, seeds and most importantly (which are removed in refined and processed carbohydrates), the outer grain coating and skins. Bran is a perfect form of fibre. You can add nuts to your cereal (keep the skins on though, to keep the goodness) in the morning to get more fibre. Soluble fibre, like bran (can be broken down easily in water) aids digestion because it is easily broken down and helps to clear your system by pushing other food through your digestive system.

Your energy level and the Glycaemic index

It's important to be aware of the types of foods that you eat, especially sugar and sugar levels, as it is this, your body fuel that directly affects your emotional state, well being and mood as well as your fat levels and appearance. One way of becoming aware of sugar levels in food is to take a look at the Glycaemic Index. You will start to see a correlation in your various energy levels and the different types of foods on it. The Glycaemic Index was originally used to help diabetics control their blood sugar levels and it can also give you a rough idea of the types of carbohydrates and sugar levels that you consume and the level of "goodness" contained within them. The scale basically measures carbohydrates and how they affect your blood sugar level and thus, your insulin level. The higher the "GI" value on the index, the more it releases sugar, at a quicker rate into the blood stream, which in turn raises your insulin levels. It is your insulin and sugar levels that drastically affect your long and short term health as well as your daily energy level. You may start to notice that if you eat lots of food from the upper end of the scale that you do not feel a sustained release of energy to help you through your day, but have an erratic energy level. You will also be suffering from exceptionally high insulin production and blood sugar levels, which is a health risk. As always, moderation is the key. Some diets also encourage you to eat high amounts of carbohydrates and low amounts of fat; again, this is not healthy. Although you may seem to lose weight, this is only a short term fix and will damage your health and body in the long term and not give you what you need to live at your optimum level, because it will increase your insulin and blood sugar level too.

I strongly encourage you to get a copy of the Glycaemic index, which you can easily find online or from your local GP. Below is a selection of foods with various "GI" levels, to give you a rough idea. It's important that you remember that these foods and their "GI" level will directly affect your energy levels and emotional state… the old saying, "you are what you eat" does indeed have a lot of truth in it.

Foods with a very high GI level

Most processed Cereals (cornflakes, for example)
White bread
White rice

Juice

Sweets

Mangoes

Raisins

Foods with a high GI level

Cake

Some biscuits

Baked Beans

Pasta

Potatoes

Peas

Oranges

Muesli

Foods with a medium GI level

Porridge

Rye Bread

Skimmed milk

Low-fat yogurts

Barley

Brown rice

Pita Bread

Chickpeas

Lentils

Kidney beans

Apples

Beetroot

Foods with a low GI level

Fish

Seafood

Chicken and Meats

Eggs

Green vegetables

Yogurt

Milk

Cottage Cheese

Soya beans

Seed

Plums

Grape fruit

Nuts

Your body's Insulin level

Your body's insulin level is directly related to what you eat and it is very important as it not only has a major effect on your appetite but also on your body fat level as well as metabolism and other important bodily functions. The hormone is secreted by your pancreas and its most important role is to balance and regulate glucose (sugar) in your blood and body. It is Insulin that regulates the level of sugar in your blood stream. And the level is directly affected by your intake of food, because your food is broken down (digested) into blood sugar, so that it can be directly absorbed and used by the body. Funny, imagine, an apple through your veins…..I digress! The point is, is that if you eat high levels of sugar that are of no use to your body, it is still forced to secrete high levels of insulin to deal with it and absorb it into the body. A fluctuating blood level is not healthy at all and directly affects your cravings and feelings of hunger as well as your mood. The imbalance is perpetuated as your body will secrete even more insulin, which will not have the desired affect on the body as it becomes desensitised to it…and even more will be needed. Obviously this can cause diabetes, heart disease, hypoglycaemia and obesity. The main causes are unhealthy consumption of simple carbohydrates and foods that register high on the "GI" index. Also, it's interesting to note, that it is these foods which give you the least nourishment because they contain the highest levels of "empty calories", which will only fill you up temporarily and leave you feeling empty and hungry, with little nutritional value. As we have already discussed, you should try and eat complex carbohydrates because it is they that will give you real energy because they are rich in nutrients and fibre. They are the ones with a lower "GI" level and raise the blood sugar levels in a sustained more healthy way…if you want to feel great, it is these that you should be incorporating into your diet, you will see real positive changes in your mood and emotional state if you start to switch from the refined processed carbohydrates like white rice, cereals, white bread, sweets and cakes to complex carbohydrates that give you lasting goodness and improve your general well being.

Carbohydrates, your mood and well being

Your mood is directly affected by the levels of noradrenalin and serotonin in your body. These neurotransmitters have a big effect on your well being and mental state and are mainly derived from carbohydrates. Some carbohydrates, like simple carbohydrates give you a temporary high, because they quickly raise your blood sugar levels and it is this fluctuation that induces a quick burst of serotonin that might temporarily feel great. The problem is that when the insulin starts to regulate your blood level, your serotonin level will also begin to drop and you will start to feel "down" and this directly affects your mood in a negative way, which of course affects behaviour…. behaviour that will probably result in more chocolate and sweets! It's not very good, and a self perpetuating cycle that will need to be broken and can be broken. You will feel so much better if you have a sustained serotonin high; you will feel great throughout the day, without the "downs" and chocolate withdrawal symptoms, if you eat foods like turkey breast, tuna and other high protein foods which contain the essential amino acids.

Practical carbohydrate advice, give it a try!

- Try and eat foods that have a low GI level
- Stay away, as much as you can, from simple carbohydrates
- When you snack, try and snack on Vegetables and fruits that have a low GI level
- Look for foods that are naturally high in fibre like whole grains and fresh vegetables
- Mix and combine your carbohydrates with proteins and other essential fats

Proteins

Protein makes up every part of your body, including your bones, blood, skin, nails and muscles. Your body is made up of mostly water, but after that comes protein. Protein is the foundation of your body and its growth and repair mechanisms. From bones, teeth, to regeneration of tissue, it is the basic building block of your body and it also helps maintain your hormonal system as well as strengthen your immune system. It is the foundation of what makes you.

Good Protein foods

Turkey breast

Chicken breast

Tuna

Trout

Lamb

Eggs

Cottage cheese

Whey

Soya products

Sardines

Cod

I would personally advise, that for a normal healthy diet, you steer clear of the protein shakes and various types of powders and supplements, unless they are used as part of a healthy balanced diet and lifestyle and with your GP's advice. Especially those weight training who might use them as part of a special diet. Also, if you have a diet that is based on shakes and drinks, then this is very unhealthy too. You may experience short term weight loss, but they will not provide you with the essential fatty acids and calories that you need as well as running the risk of developing serious health problems. Any weight lost will probably be muscle tissue as opposed to fat, very short term, and possibly detrimental to your health.

Healthy Amino Acids

There are 23 Amino acids in the body. Protein is broken down into amino acids and absorbed into the blood so that it can be used by the body. These Amino acids form structures which form various parts and functions in the body. 8 of the 23 Amino acids are essential, and these are necessary and need to be in the food that we eat, so that they can be used as building blocks for the vital proteins in the body.

Protein and how it affects your mood and well being

Your mood and emotional state is determined by various neurotransmitters, which affect your mood and feelings greatly. They are very powerful and they are your body's "Messengers" delivering signals and messages to various parts of the body, determining how you feel at any given point. Amino acids are integral in the formation of neurotransmitters which directly change your mood. Some of the well known chemical "messages" which affect your mood, feelings and well being include;

Serotonin

Different serotonin levels in the body directly affect your mood. It is the chemical responsible for your various moods, and when you don't have enough of it, you might feel down or depressed. Your body produces serotonin using various amino acids (specifically, tryptophan) found in foods like turkey breast, bananas and fish.

Adrenaline

This hormone kicks in high stress scenarios, when you might need to react quickly and gives you what you need to react decisively.

Dopamine and Noradrenalin

Dopamine and Noradrenalin are neurotransmitters that give you the feeling of control

Acetylcholine

Acetylcholine is responsible for helping you think clearly and improving your mental awareness.

Gamma aminobutyric acid

A relaxant neurotransmitter

Practical protein advice

We need to have a diet that includes all of the essential amino acids to perform to our maximum capabilities. It is important to note that not all proteins contain them. Beans, lentils, nuts, seed and pulses, often called "incomplete proteins" as they do not. Nevertheless, a healthy combination of all types in combination with food like grain, rice or Soya will give you all the protein that your body needs. Not necessarily in the same meal together though, because you can spread it out over the day and still get the same nourishment and energy. A quick and simple way of determining how much protein to eat in your meal is to take a look at the palm of your hand. The protein in your meal should cover your palm and ideally be the same thickness too. This is quite an accurate indicator to your optimum amount of protein in a meal. You generally should eat one gram of protein for every kilogram of your body weight. A quick protein snack is the best way to get full and energised over a long period. You could try a small can of tuna, sardines or even a hard boiled egg. A really tasty option is to combine your protein with carbohydrates and essential fats, like chicken or turkey breast slices a vegetable dip or vegetable small cuts.

Other protein suggestions

- Eat lots of Oily fish like sardines, mullet, salmon and mackerel as they contain essential fatty acids (omegas 3 and 6) which will improve your general well being and prevent conditions like heart disease.
- If you're vegetarian then you have a wide variety to choose from including, cheeses (low fat), Soya products, eggs, beans, seeds, tofu and pulses. Combine grains with your source of protein in the meal to complete it. Or you could try Pasta, brown rice, wholemeal bread with chickpeas, lentils or stir fried tofu with rice or vegetables and a Soya product, for a

great protein combination.
- Try and eat protein foods that are organic and fresh. Grass fed meats and organic poultry contain more nutrients, which mean that you will get more goodness from less mass.

Fats

Not all fats are bad! You can sit down to eat a really large low fat, healthy looking meal and still feel empty afterwards and unsatisfied. It's usually at this point that we turn to a packet of crisps or a bar of chocolate to fill that gap…and as the rest of the meal was really healthy, that would be alright, right? Well, not exactly! Your body does indeed need fat. It is natural and you need to eat it. The important thing is that you eat the right fats, and the right amounts of fat…as opposed to chocolates and sweets! You will only feel satisfied and full if your body has the fuel to function at its optimum, and that fuel is derived from the essential fats, that your body needs.

Fat is a very important energy source for the body…so don't get carried away with "low fat" this and "low fat" that! Those kind souls won't tell you *what* type of fat, its "low" in, and that is the key (and the rest of the really unhealthy stuff they've packed in there…a stone in the street has "low fat", but you wouldn't eat that!). Fat is an integral part of our protective system, especially protecting our internal organs and has other important functions, like in the production of hormones oestrogen, as well as progesterone. Fat also transports these hormones around the body and carries Vitamins A, E, D and K around the body as well as other fat soluble minerals too. Fat also helps maintain your weight (the right type and amounts), because it decreases your appetite, so that you eat less, because you don't feel hungry.

Different types of fat

There are two types of fat. The first is Saturated fat, which comes from cream, butter, meat, dripping and is derived from animals. Saturated fat is very concentrated and is solid at room temperature. Then there are Unsaturated fats (polyunsaturated and monounsaturated). They come from the earth (plants, for example). Like Olive oils, vegetable oils (sunflower, rapeseed oils, safflower and flaxseed oils) as well as nut oils. That said, it can also be derived from oily fish too, like tuna, mackerel and sardines. You can tell an unsaturated fat because it is liquid at normal room temperature.

Important Fatty Acids

Your central nervous system, reproductive and immune systems are all supported by essential fatty acids that are broken down from the fat that you eat. In fact, they are so important that every cell within your body will need an appropriate amount just to function properly. The fat that you eat is broken down into fatty acids and glycerol and also protects you against illness and has lots of other important functions too. The basic molecular structure of fatty acids consists of "arms" that attach themselves to carbons and hydrogens. The crucial difference between saturated and unsaturated forms is that unsaturated fatty acids contain a slightly lower number of bonds, making them looser and hence liquid at room temperature. An unsaturated fat can artificially be saturated with hydrogen and this process is called hydrogenation, creating hydrogenated fat. It's advisable to stay away from hydrogenated fat, because the body finds it difficult to metabolise, which means that it will just be stored as visible fat. You will find hydrogenated fat in foods like, low fat spreads biscuits, pastries, cereal bars and packaged foods. The process is not good for your body as the fat is artificially changed from a liquid into a solid by adding hydrogen, turning it into a semi solid. Yes…that's the stuff you eat! It has been said that this stuff can cause Cancer, birth disorders, heart disease and even low testosterone in men. You'll find it in some spreads and margarine, as well as some vegetable oils, which directly adversely affect your body, your cholesterol levels and ability to metabolise essential fatty acids.

You can eat small amounts of saturated fat like, butter and cream but it's not a good idea or a healthy one, to eat hydrogenated fats, in fact you should try and cut them out completely from your diet. You need to include unsaturated fats into your diet and specifically more of the polyunsaturated type. Beware that hydrogenated fats are usually found (and hidden!) in foods like biscuits, breaded foods, salad crèmes, margarines, various sauces, cakes, pastries, pasties, pies and things like fish fingers, as well as a lot more. Try and stick to polyunsaturated fat (or at least include unsaturated fats into your diet), and stay well away from hydrogenated fats Unsaturated fats, and specifically polyunsaturated contains two very important essential fatty acids, Omega 3 and Omega 6. Omega 3 and Omega 6 are recommended to be consumed on a very regular basis. They are great for keeping your weight down, because they act as natural indicators, preventing you from feeling the need to eat more than necessary and they produce cholecystokinin which also tells the brain that you are satisfied and full, so you don't even feel the need to overeat, or want to. They also help in burning fat so that it is not stored up visibly. That fat is used as energy so that you feel great, as opposed to round the belly, which doesn't feel so great! Omega 3 also has a positive affect on insulin in the body and in blood regulation. You can find polyunsaturated fat in oily fish, which are very good for you, like sardines, mackerel as well as in grains, nuts, vegetables, seeds and also hempseed oil and flaxseed oil.

Practical fat advice

- Include oily fish into your diet
- Eat foods that contain unsaturated fats
- Use Olive oil for cooking
- Try not to heat oils as they tend to lose nutritional value
- Instead of frying foods, why not try and grill, boil or bake.
- When you buy meat, try and buy lean organic meat/poultry
- Get rid of all hydrogenated fats in your diet!
- Try not to eat processed foods and takeaways like
- Hamburgers and fries, fish and chips, curries etc

- If you like curries then go for lamb tikka, a dry dish or chicken tandoori
- Eat oils that contain essential fatty acids like omega 3 and 6 and add them to your salad and dressings. Try lemon juice, red or white wine vinegar or garlic instead of butter. Try and add flaxseed, olive, or hempseed oil to your vegetables instead of other spreads.
- When you buy oil make sure that you keep the cap screwed on tightly so that it is air tight. Keep them in a cool dark place like the fridge, and try and purchase glass containers that are dark. Flaxseed oil should be kept refrigerated at all times

How to feel energized!

A lot of people comment on my energy level. People say that when they're around me that they themselves feel energized! Energy! I feel energized just saying the word...ENERGY! When Michael Jackson's music is on the energy just comes...and bam!!! The moves flow! But what is energy and how do I get more of it?

Energy is excitement! We've all seen Michael Jackson dance, and think wow! We can feel his energy. One man sending an audience of 100,000 into a frenzy! Now that's energy. Now…We all love to meet energetic (sane!) people. Energetic people are attractive, you want to be around them…They give you something…They can raise your spirits when your down or had a long day at work or just aren't in the mood. They give you something. Just in the same way as negative, tired people usually drain your energy and can make you feel bad. Negative energy spreads….Positive energy spreads, we all have the ability to affect other people and to determine how people see us and ultimately treat us too!

Have you noticed that if you smile, people usually smile back at you? Also, when you're feeling down have you ever tried smiling (I know it might sound crazy…But it works!). Just the physical action alone can cause a positive emotional response. It's called positive thinking, and it works, but the key factor in all of this is your Physical body…How do you actually feel? With your personal development it's important that you're honest with yourself. It's quite easy to fool the world and yourself into thinking anything, but at the end of the day positive personal growth will come with honesty and logical steps.

Some people seem really happy and energetic on the surface and look great but inside are feeling drained, over worked, over stretched and running on empty. This is actually very common... Feeling tired all the time, like you never get enough sleep and you're always working.

How do I change that?

Start with your body! Implement what you've read and you will see your energy level transform!

Summary

Water, Food, Exercise and Sleep

Drink Water. Water is the body's most important nutrient. If you do not drink enough water your body will begin to retain water as an emergency measure and you'll dehydrate. Even mild dehydration can sap your energy and make you tired. Did you know that the body can survive for up to 5 weeks without food but only 5 days without water? The minimum recommendation of water intake is 8 glasses per day and twice that for active individuals. Drink water as much as possible and as frequently as possible…You should be sipping water as you're reading this! If you want to feel energized then drink a glass of water as soon as you wake in the morning…One of those big ones…Gulp that thing down! It's a quick and easy way to get your day going in a healthy and energised way. Similarly, gulp a glass down before you go to bed too. Think about it. During your time in bed your body is using up your water supply to regulate your body's temperature as well as continue to provide the fluid environment for normal cell metabolism, turgor (structure and form of the body), sweat…. It's important to replenish your supply as soon as possible. Increase your water intake and you'll see higher energy levels through out the day. Tip: Make sure that it is clean, clear water! (Room temperature is best and tap water is fine) Beer, Wine, Vodka and Pepsi etc…Don't count!

You are made up of 60% water, which is two thirds of your body. Your brain is made of 50% water. Small changes in your fluid intake can have drastic positive effects on your well being and quality of life. Water is vital to the intracellular and extracellular functioning of your body (inside your cells, and outside, like in your saliva and blood plasma) and it's also found in vegetables and fruits (which contain about 90 percent water). Not only will water cleanse your body of all the waste materials and metabolic residual, it will give you a full "satisfied" feeling if you have a glass before your meal, as well as after. Water is absolutely calorie free, but don't be fooled by all of the various bottled "water" and sweetened drinks that usually have a lot of sugar added to them and are calorie packed (usually with pure sugar).

A very good way to see if you are drinking enough water is to take a look at your urine when you go to the toilet. It should be clear and colourless. It is essential to drink water, especially before, during and after dancing and exercise, you need to keep hydrated. You tend to perspire a lot when you exercise (as well as naturally through the day) and this can lead to fatigue and dehydration. This is easily combated by drinking lots of water. Although I recommend pure water, you can also drink fruit teas, herbal teas as well as some diluted juices. If you work in an office then you should keep a big bottle of water under your table all day and cut down on the coffee. Coffee, a stimulant and a diuretic is full of caffeine and actually pushes water out of your body, like alcohol, which is a packed carbohydrate and full of empty calories.

- Keep Alcohol and coffee to a minimum.
- Invest in a filter or purchase bottled water, if possible
- Drink 8 or more glasses of water per day
- If you drink pure fruit juices (from concentrate), why not try diluting them with water?
- Keep alcohol to a minimum. Try not to drink more than one or two glasses of wine per day.
- Why not investigate the delicious variety of fresh vegetable juices that are out there? Carrot juice is one of my favourites, and extremely tasty and healthy!
- Green teas, are said to aid weight loss, by speeding up the body's burning of fat. Drink it in moderation though because it does contain caffeine.

Healthy eating

We have all heard the saying "you are what you eat"....now that saying is exactly right! I mean you wouldn't expect your car to run efficiently without petrol, so you'd expect that we all need our "petrol" too, and to run at our best we need the good stuff! Basically, that means a healthy balanced diet, and it's essential for good health, high energy levels and for you to work (and play) at your optimum level. The key word is BALANCED.

Eating the right amounts of proteins, carbohydrates and fats in your meals will not only leave you feeling energized throughout the day but also naturally speeds up the fat burning process...In plain English: you can get into shape quicker, without the need for quick fixes crack pot dieting schemes! Balanced meals cause a hormonal response within the body, which results in burning stored body fat....Which is good news for people who like to eat "normal" food....Although as you'd expect...moderation is key also! I've already outlined what types of food is good to eat, so feel free to go through and underline and pick and choose what you feel is right for you. It's only important that you take care of the basics. There is no need for a strict health regime, with no room for enjoyment.

Enjoy plenty of whole grains, fruits and vegetables, Eat regular meals Remember to eat 5 portions of fruit or vegetables every day and to keep your intake of fizzy drinks, crisps and sweets to a minimum Eat breakfast! Eat breakfast! Quite simple and easy to enjoy.

What should we eat? A Summary

We are all different types of people with different metabolic rates. We are all unique and what works for one may not necessarily work for all, so it is important that you discover what works for you and what you feel doesn't. I'm going to summarise what we've been through and it's really important to take note if you are tempted by all of the crazy diets out there, especially the low-fat, high carbohydrates diets or the other temporary quick fix diets that can seriously damage your health. It's really quite simple. Moderation is the key to a healthy body. A healthy balance of carbohydrates, proteins and essential fats are essential for a successful healthy body and person, with lots of energy! It might take a little effort to focus and think about the foods which you consume, but the reward in the improvement of your quality of life will be worth it. It is also a decision that you choose to make, to live in a healthy way, and turn away from quick fixes that don't work. It's a worthwhile lifestyle choice that you have to make for yourself.

Try and eat foods that rate low on the "GI" scale and increase your fruit and vegetable intake, for a better source of carbohydrate.

Eat a healthy moderation of grains too. If you choose foods that rate low on the "GI" index, as part of a balanced diet, you will find yourself feeling full and satisfied a lot more, with high energy. Try and increase your protein intake, which you can get from a balanced amount of meat, fish and eggs. A palm sized amount of complete protein with each meal, and try and eat fish at least three times a week, especially oily fish with Omega 3 and 6. This will help you to feel full and satisfied and will increase your cells sensitivity to insulin.

If you want to lose weight, make sure that you eat foods that have a low "GI" and are high in fibre, so that you feel full. It's important that insulin and energy is released slowly in your body, and this feeling of well being can be attained by combining carbohydrates and proteins with a small amount of healthy fat. Eat when you feel hungry and stop when you are feeling full. If you have a snack then try and combine carbohydrates, fats and proteins, like vegetable sticks and healthy dips, nuts, meat and vegetables. Forget counting calories, as you will get all you need and have an overall feeling of well being, as well as keep your weight down by eating a common sense balanced diet. If you do cut your calories then you may feel tired throughout the day, as you're not getting the goodness you need and your metabolism may slow down. If you feel the need to eat, eat; just think about what kind of food you eat…that is the key. You can eat fat; just make sure that it's the right kind. Try and keep away from saturated fat, but try olive oils, safflower and flaxseed oils. If you're one who especially craves chocolate or sweets, you can solve that by incorporating low GI foods into your diet, as well. Finally if you have any metabolic problems or concerns about your health then immediately book an appointment and go and have a chat with your local GP or an accredited nutritionist who will be able to give you suitable advice catered to suit your needs especially if you have intolerance to certain foods etc.

General Fitness

Exercise can be fun! And it's essential that you exercise regularly so that you can keep in shape as well as feel amazing! It doesn't have to be boring or even in a gym (or dance studio for that matter!) There are many, many ways to keep fit and dancing is just one of many that are great, a lot of fun, and stimulating for the mind as well as body. You need to exercise to keep your body functioning to it's optimum level. It boosts your metabolism, keeps your stress levels down and keeps you in great shape, Your state of mind will be drastically altered for the better. Regular exercise gives you a natural high and promotes a healthy lifestyle that will be reflected in your appearance and enjoyment of life. Again, it's a case of making a conscious decision to change your life for the better. You will have to commit to regular exercise and keep at it, to see real results and you will get better at it, and enjoy it more, the more you do it and keep it up. Dancing is the best way to keep in shape in my opinion! It's fun, and you burn lots of calories and will give your body tone, especially your legs. It doesn't matter what style either. As long as your moving to the music. In fact try no style at all! As long as you're moving your body then that is a great start and a great way to keep in shape! One hour of dancing can burn about 350 calories…and you can smile while you're at it too!

Looking great!

It's important that if you want to look trim, that you burn calories so that you get rid of any excess body fat. The more you exercise, the more you boost your metabolic rate, which is the rate that you burn energy.

Your body's make up

The more muscle you have the more calories you will burn and your muscles are metabolically active even when you're relaxing. Men, usually have a higher metabolism than women because they have bigger muscles (generally). Inactivity is the killer. If you want to keep fit, then you have to perpetuate your youth by exercising! Your metabolic rate peaks in the early 20's and gently declines after that, until at around 30 years old, you start to lose muscle mass and your body fat might increase at a quicker rate…so it's important to keep exercising! If you don't, then your muscles will lose their shape and decrease in size too. This can be combated by regular, natural exercise, and you'll feel great in no time.

Ways of becoming more active. Easy ways of boosting your metabolism:

- Put your music on loud, and dance around the house!
- Walk, walk, walk! Do you really need to drive locally? If you do, be aware of where you park the car and try and park at the furthest part of the car park so that you can walk and get some exercise that way.

- Save your pound coin, dash the trolley and try carrying the shopping to the car.
- Invest in a pair of comfortable trainer (sneakers)
- Get a bicycle…it's a real investment!
- A very good way to keep fit is to stop taking the escalators and lifts; take the stairs! This is great for your legs and will get easier the more you do it
- After you've eaten, why not go out for a quick brisk walk?
- Get active…leave the remote control and jump up and change the channel manually!
- Housework can help you burn up 170 calories per hour! Make sure you pump the music up and clean with big movements, keep to the rhythm too!
- Become more active by walking and moving about more, and not being lazy! Swap automatic for manual (like lawnmowers for example)

See, you can improve your health by making small easy changes that don't involve a lot of conscious effort…and small changes like this can make a lot of difference to your health and lifestyle. It's a good start, if you want to start somewhere.

Dance and Aerobic fitness

If you want to improve your aerobic fitness and overall well being then you'll have to start using the big muscles in your body and get them moving, with large movements…dancing is perfect, but not the only way to do it! Your aerobic fitness is your ability to deliver oxygen to your working muscles and the cardiovascular system's ability to do it with ease. The more you do it, the better you will get at it and the better you will feel. You will get a metabolic boost, as your body and muscles encourage your heart and lungs to work harder and faster, to keep up with your demand. With regular exercise, you'll become naturally toned and burn fat naturally and effectively and start to look and feel great!

Aerobic exercise will improve your physicality, your well being, your appearance and benefit your lungs, give you a stronger heart and lungs, improve your posture and composure, release and relieve stress, give you psychological well being, stronger bones and so much more! Aerobic exercise is very important and it should be regular, with at least 3 thirty minute sessions per week. It's also important that it is high intensity that you focus on what you are doing and your muscles. This may be a quick walk for some people, but a fast running or sprint workout for another. It is relative, but a great indicator is your sweat levels…you need to sweat. Dancing is the perfect aerobic activity because not only does it give you a great physical workout, but also a mental workout. It really does get easier as you do it, and as we've already looked at previously, it's never usually a physical issue in the real world which prevents advancement in dance or in any physical activity, but mental barriers that can be removed with a little effort. So, in the words of Nike, "Just do it!".

Part 3: Dance and physical expression

Capturing the beauty of nature to enhance your dance and movement aesthetically

"All the world's a stage,
And all the men and women merely players:
They have their exits and their entrances;
And one man in his time plays many parts"
William Shakespeare

Don't worry about the title of the chapter...all shall be explained! When I look at a piece of choreography or any movement at all I look specifically at the shape of the body, and the manner in which certain movements are executed. If you think about it, even something as simple as walking down the street, turning to wave at your friend and then stopping for a quick chat is a pretty complex piece of choreography (when you break it down). Importantly, it is completely natural. You would never think twice about the way in which the manoeuvre was executed because it would be completely second nature to you. You would not have to think consciously about breaking down each step that you took; the way in which you stealthily pivoted on your heel for the turn and the swift raised arm that you coincided perfectly with the drop of your head and a smile. Completely natural, perfectly rhythmic and totally a piece of choreography.

What makes a "good" dance move "good" and a "bad" dance move "bad"?

I would say that there is indeed a universal law that links movement and its execution, to what is judged to be, aesthetically pleasing. In fact it is quite obvious to me that we Artists must utilise "the law", first with understanding and then with the application of it to the dance and choreography- or any other type of movement, form of human expression or art. As a result we can capture that magic that permeates through our whole existence. Both through the physical world as well as purposefully, through great art and architecture for thousands, if not millions of years. Essentially, I am talking about GEOMETRY, LINES and MATHEMATICS and how this applies to AESTETICS, STANCE, POISE. MAJESTY: A perfectly executed dance move that is pleasing to the eye, to the dancer, to the choreographer and captivates the observer by its natural elegance and beauty. The key is to try and understand WHAT makes the artistic piece so aesthetically pleasing. Is it a coincidence? Probability? Random chaos? Or is it linked to some kind of universal law or force? In relation to your body and dance it's important to be aware of what I like to call your "Body lines". "Body lines" incorporate the idea that the beauty of the choreography or movement should be conveyed through positioning and elegant execution of moves along with your natural body lines, and within certain geometric parameters, that exist and have already been studied for thousands of years, and adjudged to be aesthetically pleasing.

Now is not the time to go into depth, but I will highlight two important lines of the body that you should be aware of and the importance of working within them and also how that awareness can transform your physicality and dancing ability. I am essentially talking about proportion and certain geometric ratios such as the "Golden Ratio" or "Divine proportion" as the Ancient Greeks called it, or "Fibonacci", after the Italian Mathematician, Leonardo of Pisa. It is important that you become aware of your body and its "lines", as well as how to implement a dance step "through" those lines. At the very least, the fact that you are aware of your body will translate quite clearly in your poise and physicality. At the end of the day, you are a mover and you may want to be a dancer. It follows that you are using your body and therefore it is important to understand your physicality so that you can utilise shape and form in your dance. Shape and form are what dance and expression are all about.

I remember exactly when proportion and its relation to the human body came to my attention. I was about Seven years old and captivated by a picture that I didn't understand at the time, but knew that it was very interesting. Leonardo Da Vinci's drawing "Vitruvian Man" intrigued me even then and still does, even more so, now. He understood the body and its "lines", the aesthetic beauty contained in the very specific geometry and how that can be translated into art, and does indeed flow through all of nature. I say that a dancer should utilise this knowledge even at a basic level; flowing "through" the lines while executing any given move and at the very least appreciate the beauty of the human body.

A wonky building, with uneven sides not only looks wrong but will eventually fall, but a solid geometrical shape will remain strong and always retain a certain beauty that is clear to see. Dance is no different; I do not differentiate between human physical movement to rhythm and the various kinds of sacred architecture or great art, from the Renaissance or any other time in history, which are quite obviously linked to sacred and complex mathematical ratios and the geometry hidden within. In fact as a choreographer, I feel that the "sacred geometry" that is observed throughout the universe, which has been understood and incorporated into Art by numerous great philosophers and Artists, should be all the more observed and incorporated in varying degrees, into dance. At that stage, we shall indeed see magic and the power of the body as well as the spirit manifesting in a truly glorious performance.

What is "Divine proportion" and how does it relate to dance and movement?

Well, "Phi" is a sound and the 21st letter of the Greek alphabet; it is a number (1.618...), but specifically a very important number with unique properties. It is a number and proportion which Renaissance artists called "Divine Proportion". The mathematician Luca Pacioli published *"De Divina Proportione"* in 1509, where he investigated and explored the relationship between mathematical proportion and the visually stimulating and aesthetically pleasing. He was a trained artist and a friend of Leonardo Da Vinci. The book had a massive influence on future artists, architects and those interested in visual expression. It was Leonardo Da Vinci who seemed to promote the idea that the human body was also linked to the Golden Ratio, he also illustrated the book. It is clear, although keenly debated, that he incorporated it in his other works, like the Mona Lisa and other amazing pieces that are known for their amazing beauty. It is likely that he and other great artists before him, as well as since (Mondrian and Salvador Dalí for example) have proportioned their Art, Paintings, sculpture, architecture and man made beauty according to the golden ratio and other proportions. Interestingly, the golden ratio proportion can be seen in many of the most magnificent and beautiful creations ever constructed. The Egyptians used it in the creation of the pyramids. The Ancient Greeks were guided by it in the construction of the Acropolis and it was also used later in the design of the Notre Dame Cathedral in Paris.

Whatever this "magic proportion" is, it is not only restricted to man made objects. It is found in nature, throughout the human body, plants, space and the proportions of the planets, music and the Arts and throughout the whole universe. The German intellectual Adolph Zeising (1810-1876) who researched exhaustively into the link between the golden ratio and man made objects as well as in nature wrote, in 1854;

"[A universal law] in which is contained the ground-principle of all formative striving for beauty and completeness in the realms of both nature and art, and which permeates, as a paramount spiritual ideal, all structures, forms and proportions, whether cosmic or individual, organic or inorganic, acoustic or optical; which finds its fullest realization, however, in the human form"

It is quite clear that aesthetical beauty and geometric proportion are linked in a very special way, some might even say in a spiritual way. The initiated have propagated this through masterpieces for centuries and I am in total agreement. Form and proportion are fundamentals in dance and it is essential that in conveying real artistic beauty, this is not forgotten. It is not only an integral part in an artistic sense but also in a way of maximising and utilising strength too. Stance has always been important; we just need to take a look toward the east and the various martial arts to get a sense of that. The "Hachiji dachi" stance in Karate is based on the Kanji; the shape for the number 8, in Japanese writing and it is thought to specifically maximise strength. This is very important to grasp. A certain stance or position maximises your physical strength and ability to "perform" the next step effectively. It is also believed by some, that certain stances also enhance the spirit and allow it to flow freely through the movement.

Any great artist in History, from Michael Jackson to Leonardo Da Vinci to John Lennon has spoken about this in other ways, they often expressed that they were just vessels and that the magic just flowed into them and through them, and that they were there to capture it at that particular time. The key is to be available at the time and to be accepting of the magic when it does eventually arrive! It's also very important that you, as the reader, understand that the great artists do not think in categories and boxes. Something that is aesthetically beautiful is beautiful; whatever label you want to place on it, a great piece of music is a great piece of music, no matter what you want to call it. Likewise an amazing piece of choreography, a karate stance, or the poise of a leopard, before it attacks or even the design of a building are all beautiful physical expressions. It is that simple. They are all linked. The labels that we give different kinds of physical expression usually serve to divide us from them, or at the very least, serve as a psychological divide, that can prevent us from appreciating them or taking a look and considering them in the first place.

It's quite interesting that a "label", like a "value", is just an idea. Nothing more, an idea in someone's head…and quite usually a barrier…which is interesting when you think about it. Imagine the freedom, enjoyment and experience that might be gained if we dropped a lot of them and just absorbed and appreciated things as they really were, good or bad, right or wrong.

Let's take a look at a couple of examples. One of the most frequent questions that I get asked as a choreographer is, "What style do you dance?" Now, that is a very interesting question, because the short answer should be "any style that I choose, at any given time". If I choose to take a ballet step and incorporate it with a hip hop step, and then change the dynamics of the piece by fusing it with a spice of jazz and pinch a few of the swinging upper arm movements from the masked native American Indians in Alaska. What do you call that style? Why does it need a name in the first place? I will give it a try, without fear or restricting labels or names (in somebody else's head) and if it works then great…and if not, no big deal! We are free to express ourselves!

On the other hand, one might find the greatest urban street dancer on the planet, right in the middle of the city and try and convey the beauty of a Demi-Pointe to him without success due to the stigma attached to Ballet in that particular location. It is when great minds do start to think outside the box, without the labels and prejudices, that amazing ground breaking human expressions start to happen.

Just think of the moonwalk! Think about it, what is the moonwalk composed of exactly? A fusion of Demi- Pointe and a raw slide from the street, perhaps? Again, somebody must have just tried it out and had a unique idea. Michael Jackson too, for example, fuses every style out there in his short movies! You might have a jazz dancer who watches Michael dance in "The way you make me feel" or "Beat it" and say to themselves "I could never do that", but in actual fact, every step from those two particular videos was derived directly from the Jazz/Ballet Broadway musical "West Side Story". Yes…Every choreographed step! Now that same dancer would have no difficulty at all with the steps from West Side Story. Now that is not logical at all! Again, the problem arises, not from the reality of the situation and the dancer's actual ability, but from the dancer's mind and from the application of labels.

Dance & physical expression   131

These labels prevent honest consideration, simple learning and simply executing the moves.

I'll say it again: great artists and thinkers do not think in terms of categories or labels! They are merely marketing ploys, most of the time anyway! A commercial initiative separate from the Art, as a means of reaching (a polite way of saying "selling" to!) more people who are only comfortable consuming in the average pigeon hole way. It should be irrelevant to the artist or thinker as it often prevents artistic growth (or just human growth for that matter!). If you think or attempt to create with the shackles of self restriction you will never reach your full potential. You have capped your talent level from the outset: the main point of this book!

You may be getting my point already…I do not differentiate between a choreographed dance sequence and a "random" physical reaction and movement to something in the street. The only difference between a preconceived dance step or a so called piece of choreography and a random physical action, is intention. In fact the beauty contained within that "random" unplanned set of movements has the ability to far exceed the beauty of a pre planned set of movements any day! Why? Because it is an honest natural expression of who we are, without the conscious fear, doubt and restriction that we as people in this system place upon ourselves everyday.

The key word is "honesty", followed by "natural". Nature and the natural are where beauty lies. If you've ever observed the amazing herds of wilder beast in Africa and various animals or a flock of birds migrating, you'd be awestruck by the seemingly choreographed totally cohesive movement and "dance" that is performed. Literal perfection and beauty that we humans can only aspire to reproduce on the stage or in any artistic capacity. That said, it is interesting that a herd by definition is unstructured; however, if you look closely at the movement and observe, you might just notice a few leading animals. They are copied by the rest of the herd; they "choreograph" this beautiful scene and direct the others. Technically this particular animal is called the "control animal" and it is they that choreograph this natural spectacle. It is a truly amazing feat. Would it be too much, I ask to study the movements of wilder beast or flying birds and incorporate them into your art or dance? Not at all! Why wouldn't that be one of the first places to search for inspiration in the first place?

The truly great minds have been doing this for thousands of years, because they have understood the link between nature and aesthetically pleasing man made creations. Of course, that we are natural beings that inhabit the earth and are linked to it in everyway is especially relevant. I would also highlight the bridge between what we view as "out there" or as "irrelevant to us", for it might sometimes be a lot more significant than we might imagine. We often ignore and overlook such scientific connections that are totally relevant to our growth, our art and our lives because we prejudge them away, to our loss. Even the beauty of a herd of animals is closely linked in physical movement, responses and emotional behaviour to human beings that it would certainly shock some people. Human phenomena and behaviour like fashion "fads", popular "crazes", stock market crashes, flash riots, religious movements and actions can all be attributed to involve "herd behaviour". Even down to the physical day-to-day movements of people on the tube, on the streets and around the town. All choreographed, consciously or unconsciously, all natural and all linked to wilder beasts roaming the open plains!

The natural choreography that is generally ignored is often the biggest most amazing expression, because it is unconscious. I cannot walk around any major city and not be captivated by the sequence of events around me; all this transpires into the most amazing choreographed routine (usually the same one daily, I hasten to add!) around the specifically placed landmarks, that make the stage, as Shakespeare once said! Anybody who has been to Cairo, Egypt will have observed the "magic in the madness", so to speak, and the beauty in the hustle and bustle and constant horn blowing that create a wonderful, yet very interesting, symphony of noise that you'll never forget!

This can be taken further though. I do not think that it is necessary to restrict yourself in any way at all. I do not think that it is at all essential to differentiate between any type of physical expression (or any other kind of expression) that is aesthetically pleasing (or not for that matter!). It is that conscious act of differentiation that, as well as stifling growth, might prevent us from expressing ourselves to our maximum capability before we even start to follow our idea through or our heart or our inner most dreams and desires.

Experiencing different types of supposedly unrelated forms of beauty, and as artists, interpreting them and moulding them for our audience is what a true artist can do; it is amazing what wonderful results can come from this kind of non linear thought process. It can be a real learning and educational process for all involved. YOU, the reader are the artist and the world is YOUR stage! You are free to express yourself in any way you choose, using anything or any kind of inspiration you choose, at any particular time, for any particular reason. Be it work, play, performance, relaxation, following your dreams, parachuting out of a plane! Whatever! You are free to express yourself. Don't forget that!

A musical note, a dance move, a perfectly structured building, a flower, the planets, a statue, a cat, a dog, an ocean: use them all as your inspiration. Why differentiate between them at all? Why mentally restrict yourself? You are free to think outside the box and outside of your universal schooling and training (which often only encourages linear thinking, and punishes the opposite). You have the ability to think in a non generic way, because you are a unique individual. What an amazing world of beauty, diversity and fulfilment we could live in, if we would only unlock the mental restrictions that we have placed on ourselves and walk away from them.

Diversity and seemingly unrelated things are just ideas or concepts in the head. With education and additional information considered, something that might seem unrelated or irrelevant to you might in actual fact, change your whole way of thinking and quality of life or direction. Which might have been left unconsidered, or undiscovered due to ignorance or the simple lack of knowledge and understanding. I would say that it's important to free yourself and realise that not only can you learn from all, and incorporate seemingly diverse and unrelated things together as one expression of physical beauty, but if you choose to do so then that is when you will find the most unique kind of fulfilment and magic. True Art!

Expression is expression and you are free to utilise the lot, in your own unique way, if you choose. The American choreographer Wade J Robson, an amazing talent understood this when he studied the birds migrating. He observed their natural grace and incorporated the movements into his choreography and dance. The pioneer of electronic music, Jean Michel Jarre, understood this when he explained that there is no difference between a sound (e.g. rain hitting the window, a hammer hitting a nail or a car starting) and a "musical note", except for the artist's intention.

You are free to express yourself and take inspiration from anywhere you choose.

One of my favourite pieces of choreography is from Michael Jackson's History world tour and the performance of his hit song "They don't care about us". It is a montage of various styles but the under-pinning theme is a military one. The rebellious nature of the song is reinforced with a thumping drum cadence, the kind of rhythms and beats that have obviously inspired Michael and Janet Jackson through the years and impressed audiences around the world. The emphatic force, military style and swift movement is unique, inspired and a joy to watch. They recreate that aggression live on stage with the simplicity of the moves in perfect conjunction with the driving beat. Where did the inspiration for this powerful piece of choreography come from? Well, it would seem to me, that it was inspired by a very interesting place indeed. Malaysia…and specifically the Malaysian riot police! The first time I saw it, I knew straight away and noticed the marching simultaneously timed with the raising of the right arm against the left shoulder forcefully, and the slamming of the leg and arm back down, all in unison; it was borrowed from a very unique place.

The Malaysians are known to crack down swiftly on any kind of civil disobedience and they do so with a show of brute force and intimidation. To disperse a crowd they send in the riot police in full gear and a shield in their left hand and a baton in their right hand. While marching forwards in unison, a soldier raises up his baton, in perfect time with his left leg and brings it down thunderously, striking the left hand side of his shield. It is a very loud and intimidating show of military force, but at the same time a rhythmic and choreographed wonder. Tap into that power and incorporate it into a live concert setting to convey a feeling of aggression to the audience - this equals true genius, in my opinion! This sentiment is echoed by the audience reaction and world wide acclaim of the King of Pop, and respect for his uniqueness and vision!

It is that vision and ability to search and be inspired by the seemingly unrelated, that you too have; vision that should be free, clear, unfiltered and available to be inspired from all areas and aspects of life without prejudice. It's just a case of unlocking and allowing yourself to think freely…quite simple! You'd be surprised at what you can achieve and the directions that you can travel when you remove the barriers, take away the learned filters and just go with your inner feelings and intuition. I'm not exclusively talking in an artistic sense either; you can apply that same mind set to all aspects of your life.

What is "dance" exactly and how do I enhance it?

Before we take a closer look at ways to improve our dance and movement ability and think about ways to enhance the aesthetic nature of it, I think that it's important to first define and then examine exactly what the word "dance" means. Technically the word is an expression of human physical movement in a variety of different settings (i.e. performance, social, spiritual) and more precisely is a method of non-verbal communication. It's important to note that dance and music (sound and rhythm) have an obvious symbiotic relationship, and for that reason I try not to differentiate between them as forms of expression too often. Now, a key word is movement, which is defined in the dictionary as "the act, process, or result of moving" and even more relevant to us right now, "a particular manner or style of moving", which is simple enough. The usual problem is the manner and style of the movement and how it is interpreted and what differentiates a classy stylised move to a drunken attempt at the same thing!

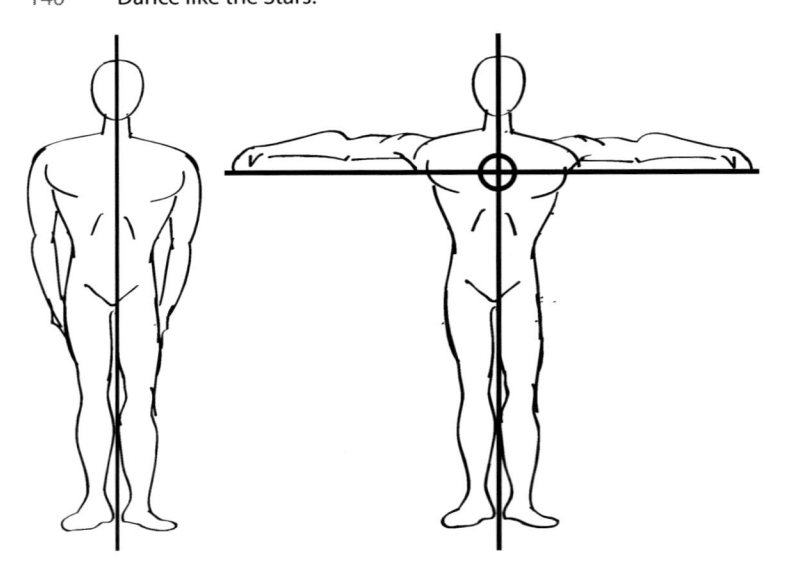

So, it's clear that movement is just motion from point A to point B in an aesthetically pleasing or stylised way. But what exactly makes the move aesthetically pleasing or at least a tolerable physical expression that has some kind of form and that simply put: looks good? I would say that *style, form, poise, consistency, timing, placement, control* and *accuracy* are at the top of list and all make up the concept of aesthetically pleasing execution of movement, in the physical sense. Let's first take a closer look at some of these things and the reasons why it is important to be aware of them and implement some simple techniques to improve them.

Any performer or person who is aware of their own anatomy is in a position of control and can utilise their body in a better way than somebody who is not. It's clear to see when somebody doesn't have this awareness, they may be off balanced or look uncomfortable. I also think that it is not important for us all to be experts in anatomy or the optimal balance of weight in our body movements, but the fact that we have a cursory understanding and awareness, will help balance and positioning. Just the idea of thinking about your body, standing up straight, head up or executing a movement through a line, will indeed translate to better physicality.

As you can see from the diagrams, your body is made up of lines and it is important that you are aware of them. When you are executing a dance move, think about executing it along the full length consistently, while keeping strictly within the line. The most important line in the body is your centre line (vertical) and secondly your horizontal line through your sternum and arms.

When thinking about our physicality and position the most important aspect is our spine. This means we stand up straight with our head up. Any movement should originate from that centre line consistently, unless a step is intended otherwise. It's also important to be aware of your sternum. If you are going to swing your arm to the left, after raising it up, for example, it should originate at the sternum to the left, with a consistent speed, and across and through the line (as outlined in the diagram) without wandering from it (unless it is intended otherwise). The start point of any movement is of importance, as is the end point. Some seem to forget that it is the whole movement that is judged. Keep any movement inside your lines (see diagrams), but be aware of the start and end point also. If that start or end point is kept within your obvious straight lines, without wandering out, and is executed with consistency, then it should look great. If you wander from (unless you intend to) a line, to return to it, then this will not look aesthetically pleasing, unless you intended to wander from that line or to make it look a certain way. A straight line is usually the shortest distance between the start of the movement and the end of it and if you think about the various lines in the body and focus on moving your body through them, you should remain balanced and looking great.

Poise

The dictionary definition of poise states that it is a "state of balance, equilibrium or stability" and for obvious reasons good poise is the foundation of a good dancer. Posture is where it all begins, so if you want to dance or walk down the street in a straight line, it's important to keep your back straight and lengthened.

Exercise

Find a nice straight wall and go and stand with your back up against it. It is important that you align your feet (heels), your backside (tailbone) as well as your upper back (shoulder blades) completely up against the wall so that you are completely vertical and looking straight ahead as well. This should be your default natural stance. Make sure that you are aware of your stomach and pull it in without holding your breath and using your stomach muscles. It's also important that you relax somewhat, but be aware of your spine and especially your head. Don't let it drop down. At this point you can step away from the wall, making sure that you keep the confident disposition (head up, chest up and a lengthened neck). You now have a reference for good posture and it's important that while you work on improving it you remain aware and constantly re-adjust. Another great way to do this is to place a light book on your head before you step away from the wall and try and keep balanced, while you walk away. It's important to stay focused and stay balanced. I call this exercise "PEAP": posture and poise equals aesthetically pleasing!

Style

Michael Jackson's choreographer was once asked to describe the difference between Janet and Michael's dance styles and he replied that Janet loves to "thrash" and that Michael has a certain elegance about the way he moves. I love that and agree totally. He has a certain kind of Majesty. The same that you would expect to see in a principal ballet dancer. He understands that it is not about the amount of moves you do, but in the quality and intensity of the moves that you do. In fact Michael Jackson specifically, dances very little on stage as he likes to walk around a lot. Also, importantly, he is not afraid of utilising various dance styles, from tap to street to jazz to ballet. A basic grasp of ballet and jazz is ideal for a dancer but as with verbal communication, the larger your physical dance vocabulary, the more you will be able to communicate physically, which is why it is a great idea to try as many styles as you can. You will eventually find your own unique style if you watch as many varied dancers as you can and utilise their moves. Imitation is actually the key to developing your own style. Remember the bigger your style vocabulary, the more range you will have as a dancer. Michael Jackson used to stand watching and learning from James Brown. If you imitate and dance as many styles as you can, you will eventually find your own unique style that you are comfortable with.

Timing

Correct timing is essential for any dancer. Opinions vary on what is the best way to improve your timing. Most trained choreographers will encourage you to count and some will say that it is an absolute must. My opinion differs slightly. If you are training and practicing for a piece, without accompaniment, then indeed, counting is essential and will help you keep form and improve progressively. Slow counting, out loud, gives you control and flexibility of pace as you practise. After rehearsal and practice is over though, I honestly feel that it is not necessary that you count in your head at all. As we have looked at earlier, you should almost put yourself in a state where the music flows through you. You already have your timing in the instruments. Let the snare and bass kick count for you. They are in effect metronomes; so why in addition to that would you need to count when you can trust the drums or percussion to do it quite effectively for you! Again, let the music flow through you and move with it as if you are one. A way to improve your timing is to become totally reliant on the music by becoming more familiar with it. It's surprising how much easier choreography and dancing become when you listen to the music and become an expert in the piece that you are dancing to. At the end of the day it is the music which should dictate the physical movement, use it and its count as your metronome. If you don't have music, then count, but look at it as a temporary replacement of the music rather than a framework which you can't break out of, or a supplement to the music or song. Think about it, what's the difference between rhythm and counting and which is essential out of the two? You can indeed learn to count, but to have rhythm comes from inside you and your state and confidence as well as your connection to the music.

Control

Control of your body and movement is what dancing is all about and it is essential to master your body and movements so that you look good, stay injury free and move correctly. A dancer by definition should move in a controlled manner. Adrienne Leitch, in "Dance: concise definitions of universal dance terms", puts it this way: "control - the ability to manage a variety of body actions with concentrated awareness of muscular activity in order to retain personal equilibrium". (Co-ordination) balance and control can be improved by firstly, moving slowly and secondly thinking slowly! Work methodically through each step with full consideration of poise, balance and where you intend to place your body. Other ways of improving your control are to work on your physical strength, especially your core strength and listen to the music and move with it. Think about what you are doing and execute each step in an intentionally slow way and with time you will begin to master your movement.

Placement and Accuracy

Speed is an essential part of dance, but NOT at the expense of accuracy and form. When the music is pumping and the blood is flowing it is easy to forget about your form and increase the tempo and energy you exert and put into a step. The opposite should be the case. The accents of a piece of music, for example are enhanced by the accuracy and placement and not your speed, or increased speed at the expense of control. In fact speed will increase with your confidence after you have mastered a step, but not before.

So always start slow, master your step, focus on accuracy and placement, and when the music is turned up, stay relaxed and focused rather than increase your speed or energy level. Your body posture and alignment is of utmost importance and it is essential that you remain focused on that throughout dancing and performing. Focus on keeping your body upright and eyes level as well as letting the music hit the mark, dictating your movements. The faster you execute a step the more likely you are to miss your mark. It's essential that you think about your style, form, placement, control and accuracy if you want to dance well.

Learning the Moonwalk

Although Michael Jackson hugely popularised the moonwalk, as it is known today, the step is also known as the "backslide". The moonwalk is actually a slightly different move which is a combination of floating, gliding and sliding, and has a more circular movement, which I like to call the "circle slide". Michael Jackson first showcased the moonwalk in his legendary performance of "Billie Jean" in 1983 at the Motown 25th anniversary show. But in actual fact dancers like the legendary Jeffrey Daniel, who subsequently choreographed for Michael Jackson were performing the backslide years earlier. Before that James Brown performed a kind of moonwalk but it was a street dancer called Cooley Jackson who apparently taught Michael Jackson the backslide. One of the most impressive backslides was performed in 1955 at the end of a tap sequence by the entertainer Bill Bailey. It is clear though, that although he did not invent it, it was Michael Jackson who has made the move world famous. So I think we should give it a try…here goes!

Ideally for this move you will need a smooth surface, comfortable trainers or any light shoes and comfortable clothes. Although it is ideal that you have a smooth surface to execute the moonwalk, it can be executed on carpet or pavement or any surface that doesn't have a substantially high amount of friction (like sand or mud, for example!). Pavement or less is fine. In fact I suggest that you practice on a rougher floor first to get used to the mechanics of the steps and get used to pushing and transferring the weight into the floor so that it is easier when you want to perform or show off the move on the dance floor! The illusion of this move comes from the execution of the weight transfer, accurately, as opposed to the sliding which is why the moonwalk is classed as a "popping" move and not necessarily a "glide" as it may seem.

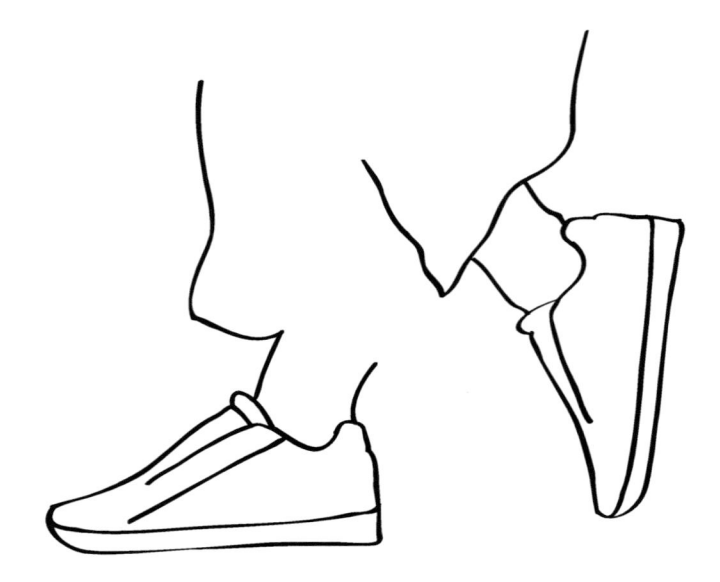

Dance & physical expression   151

Starting position: Start with your back straight and your feet together pointing forward.

Step 2: "The L position": Lift your right leg
and place the toes of your right foot down on the floor approximately a foot behind your left leg.

Try and keep a solid stance, so that you can put weight onto your back foot and toes, while keeping your "L" shape stance. You'll achieve this by varying the position of your back foot in relation to your front. If it's too close then it might be unstable. Keep a solid L shape!

Step 3: Balance: If you feel off balance you can increase the width between your legs to create a wider centre of gravity.

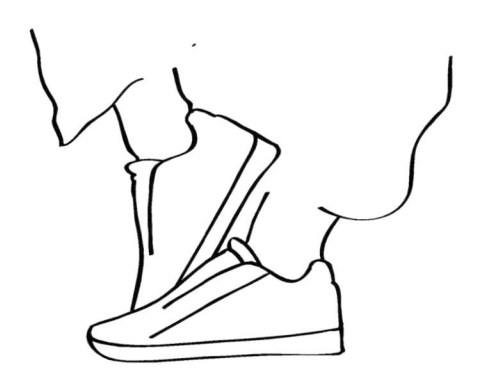

Step 4: The slide: Lean back onto your rear leg and slide the left heal back and into the floor, so that it finishes behind the right leg. At the end of the movement snap the heel of your left foot up, off the floor. It's important that you keep the heels of your feet at opposite positions and then only snap them and reverse the positions very quickly in one swift step.

The aim, is for one foot to be vertical and the other to be horizontal, and then snap, keeping the form in reverse. Only snap your heel down at the END of the movement. Although this is difficult at first, you'll get used to it.

Purposefully keep your heel upright, until it's physically impossible to sustain your L shape because of your weight transfer and heel snap while sliding, push the heel of your foot backwards but most importantly DOWN, into the floor. This is important. The pressure of your heel should push into the floor so that it is an effort to slide the foot backwards.
It is this effort that creates the illusion and the force of the snap. Really focus on pushing your heel into the floor and back rather than just dragging your foot backwards. Again, it's the up and down thinking and movement that will create the illusion of the move.

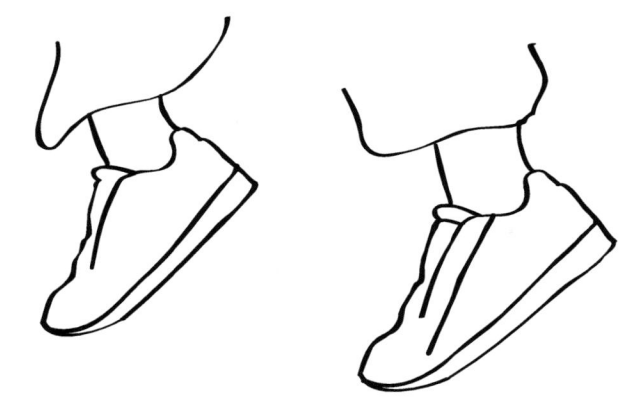

The toes of both feet should never come off the floor even if your heels do.

Step 5: The Snap: As you snap your left heel up off the floor, your right heel should simultaneously snap down on to the floor. This is a solid weight transfer, which is a very quick and heavy movement. It might help if you think of your body movement as "up and down" as opposed to "forward and back", because the weight transfer is from heel to heel and up and down. Remember to keep your back straight and head and body up right while you carry out this step.

Copy: From the finishing position of the last move duplicate the slide on the other foot. It takes time to join up the steps so that they flow. While you practice, it might make sense to pause and rest in between each step. It is an unnatural position and movement, so it takes practice and getting used to as well as getting used to strengthening your feet and toes.

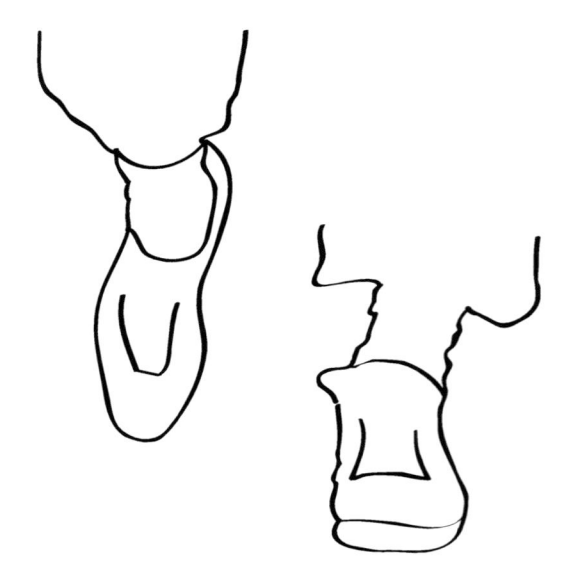

Step 6: The head: To help to create the illusion of the move, add a head movement. As you slide your leg back slowly move your head forward as if it's being left behind the movement and then pull it back towards the body as you switch to the other foot.

Really stretch your neck forwards, pushing your chin forward. If you focus on your chin and under neck area, while still keeping head up right, you'll be able to extend your head further forward. Slowly push forward and pull your neck back with speed, in sync with your legs and the snap.

Step 7 "The arms": To make the step look even better, swing your arms as if you're walking forward normally, while keeping them in time with your leg movements. As your left leg slides back your right arm should swing forward.

It might seem near impossible at first, which is completely normal. Practise the sequence a lot! It takes at least four hours of solid practising just to get used to the concept, but after practice and focusing on your form and stance, you'll be busting the step everywhere and impressing all your friends and more importantly yourself!

The side slide!

The next dance step we're going to take a look at is called a "glide". We are going to try and glide toward the side giving the illusion that we are floating on air, effortlessly. A glide is very much related to popping and is very similar to the moonwalk, but has more of an effortless, smooth quality to it. We will be using our feet to push, pull and turn to create the illusion. This move was popularised, again by Michael Jackson but has recently been attempted and varied by pop artists like Justin Timberlake and Usher, who have tried to add their own unique interpretation to the step. I personally like the smooth yet sharp quality of Michael Jackson's glide. I like to call the step the "side slide" and it is one of my favourite steps, as it is quick and easy to perform after it has been mastered. Feel free to vary it and add your own interpretation and ideas to the move.

This is essentially a street dance step and consists of pretty unnatural body movements. Which adds to the illusion, as it looks like it is impossible to do, but only adds to the surreal effect. It's important to remember to learn one step at a time.

Firstly, break down the move and isolate each component; next master each one; and later join them together. Isolation is the key to this step; that is, moving different parts of your body independently of the rest. This requires focus and practice. But after a little practice it becomes second nature - you'll start enjoying it once you've practised so much that you stop thinking about the steps, and just let your body go with the flow. As with every step or piece of choreography, try and allow the music to flow "through" you as opposed to dancing "on" the beat.

One way of doing this is to literally imagine you are part of the music or an instrument in it, like a drum. Most important is practice and methodical conditioning. So let's have a closer look at the "side slide"…

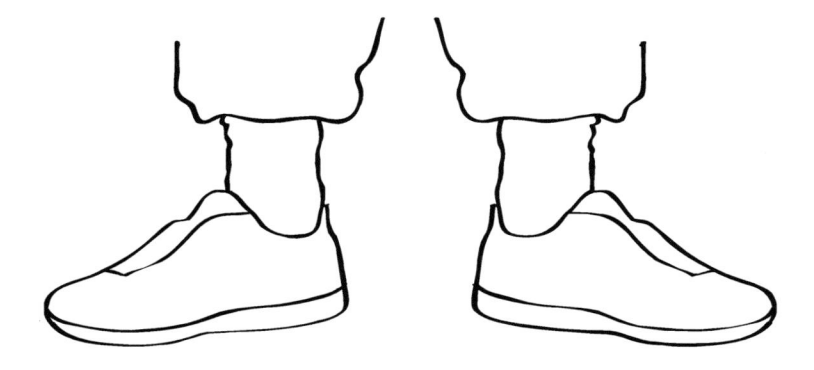

Starting position: Stand with your back straight and your chin up. Place your feet shoulder width apart pointing diagonally outwards.

- Bend your left leg at the knee and in the direction that your foot is pointing while raising your left heel off the floor. Keep your body up right and straight. You should feel the muscles in your left thigh working as they take your weight. It's important that you do not lean over. Keep your spine and upper body completely straight as you lower your self into position.
- The pivot: You're now going to pivot on your left toe and right heel so that both of your toes are pointing inwards. Transferring your weight on to the left toe, swing your left heel toward the left. The position of your toes does not move, in relation to the floor.

At the same time, transfer the weight on your right foot, on your heel, swinging your toes in and to the left, raising your toes slightly off the floor. The heel of your right foot should not move its position in relation to the floor. Pivot both feet at the same time, with speed, keeping your back straight and your knees bent, as in the previous step.

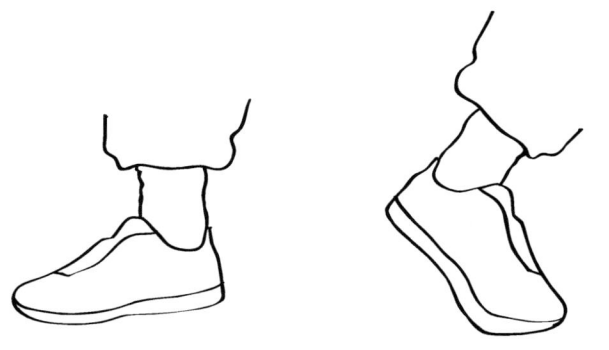

Leg snap: Your left knee will be bent and your right straight. Snap your left knee back, and your right knee forward, so that this is reversed. Your right knee should push slightly toward the left at a diagonal and your left leg should snap toward the right at a diagonal.

It's important that you keep your knees bent and back straight, as you will be tempted to straighten up. Keep the form of the first step throughout and keep low. When executing the leg snap, do not move any other part of your upper body (imagine an Elvis Presley shuffle!)

- Right angle: To prepare for the sliding motion you should turn your right heel in towards the other leg, while keeping your toe in contact with the floor. You might feel slightly unstable, temporarily, but it's important that you keep your form.

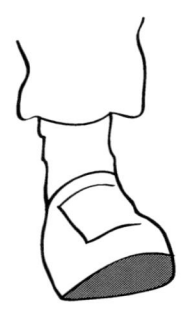

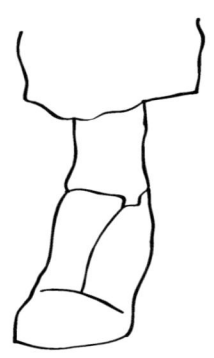

- The slide: You are now going to use your right foot to slide to the left. As you push off, turn your left foot in the direction that it is sliding and take the weight onto your left toes to stop the slide. When you push off the right foot, remember that you are to transfer equal weight off your right foot, into the left foot.

From there you should slide the foot into the floor and toward the left. You will create friction with the ground. It is that effort that will create the illusion that you are gliding. Remember to keep your back fully straightened and to transfer the weight through your legs and heels, in a snap. A "push, slide and snap (right heel down on the "snap")" motion. You might be tempted to raise up the toes of the left sliding foot, but keep them pushing into the floor and down at the same time as you slide toward the left in a swift sharp movement.

The heel drag: Drag your right heel toward your left foot while pivoting on your left toes. Your heel should slide along and into the floor in a straight line (approx 20- 30 cm). When you pivot on the left foot, remember that the position of your toes do not change in relation to the floor and you are raising up, and swinging the left, your left heel simultaneously with the heel drag on the right foot.

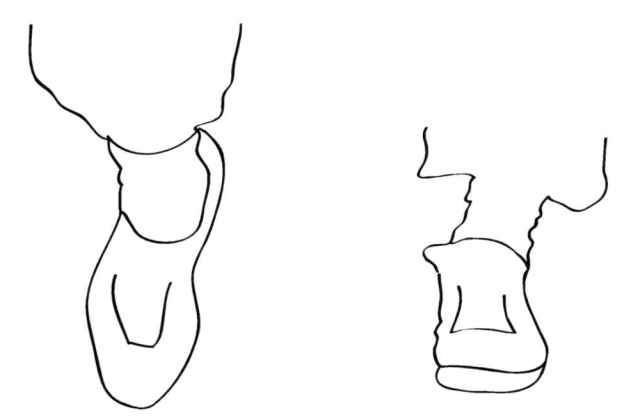

The toe flip: At the end of your heel slide, flip your right foot so that your toes are touching the floor and your heel is raised. Your foot should move in a swift movement, without moving in relation to the floor. You should imagine that you are pushing your right heel forward, while raising it, on the pointed foot. Keep it in, and tight while keeping the form of the rest of your body.

Second slide: From this position you are now going to push off into another slide. Push down and into the floor with your right foot whilst sliding your left foot away. Remember to push your left toe in the direction you are travelling and keep your back upright and straight at all times. Also keep in mind that it is an equal weight transfer via the floor! The friction and effort is a good thing, which you will get used to, but it is essential. If this is not an effort then you're sliding into the floor incorrectly and should push harder into the floor, so that it is!

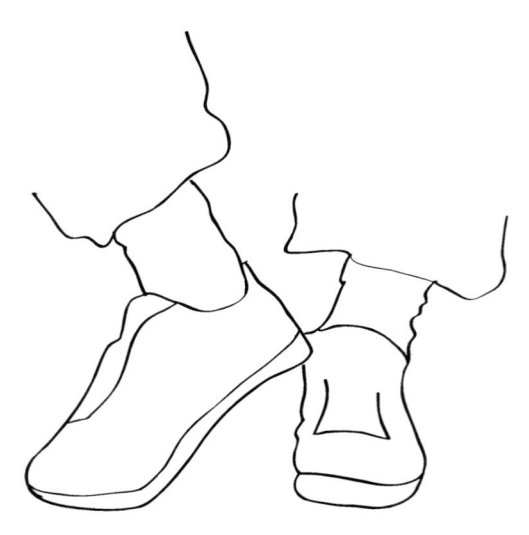

Heel drag: Repeat the heel drag as before by sliding your heel inward to the left while pivoting your left toe inwards. At the end of the movement flick your toes down and your heel up once more.

Join it up! You now have all the necessary footwork to pull the side slide off, but next you have to join it up into one continuous line by accurately repeating the moves to build up speed and smoothness. It's important that before you attempt to join it up you master each step individually as well as focusing on isolating parts of your body. So that when you pivot (for example) the step has no effect on any other part of your body or your position or stance. Throughout this move (especially when learning the mechanics of the step) it's important to remember that the movements of the legs should not have any effect on your upper body or spine and that you should stay low and keep your body relative to the ground through the steps. It's also important that you master each step before attempting to join them up, so that when you do join them up, it is a natural progression to the slide. At this stage the weight transfers should be very mechanical and you should become very aware of your weight and where you are placing it through your body. The slide works because you are using weight transfer in a very unnatural way, which creates the illusion. It takes a while to get used to. With perseverance you will get it!

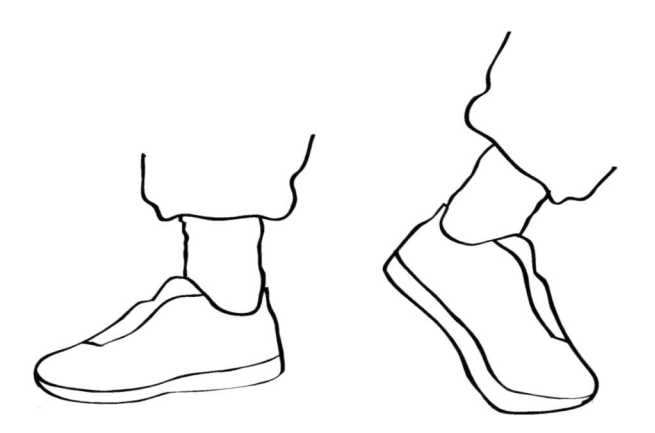

The upper body

The arms: To complete the step add some upper body movement. Keep your arms straight and bring them to the front of your body with your fingers together pointing outwards and your palms parallel to the floor. Next, move your arms up and down from the shoulder. Add in a rotation so that your arms look like pistons driving the motion through the slide and the rest of your body. Do this at the same time as you are rotating to enhance the illusion.

Dance & physical expression   165

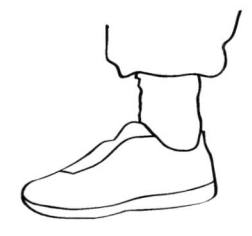

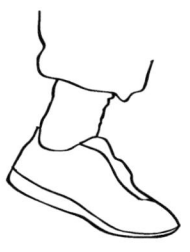

The head: Keep your back straight and make a circular movement in a clockwise direction with your head. Be careful not to jerk your neck, keeping the move smooth and steady. Really stretch your neck forwards, pushing your chin forward and down and then around in the circular motion. Focus on keeping your head completely straight, so that you do not tip in any direction. You can do this by keeping your eyes looking straight ahead and focusing on pushing the move with your chin and under neck area rather than your head. If you focus on your chin and under neck area, while still keeping your head upright, you'll be able to extend your head further forward and around in a clean simple motion, without it looking awkward.

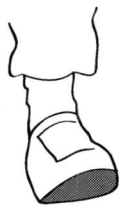

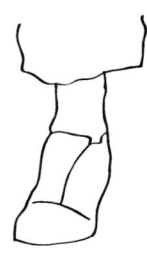

Remember, practise makes perfect! The side slide needs a lot of practice to master, but if you put the effort in and focus on each step and try to understand the mechanics of the motion…you'll soon be busting the side slide everywhere!

There is no doubt that this seems like a complicated step, but with practice and training it really does become second nature and a joy to perform and watch. As with most dance steps there will be a certain point when it just feels right and it "clicks" into place (after practice). It may seem impossible before this point, but it is so important that you focus and keep going. It is a misconception that popping and locking are difficult and that only some people are able to do it. As with everything, if you break it down and practise each step slowly, then it will come together and in the end you will be able to do it with accuracy and confidence.

For more dance tips and demonstrative videos:

www.anthony-king.com

Simple Stretching

Stretching is important and is essential for any exercise or dance program. You're stretching the muscle so that it is prepared and ready for exercise. Stretching can prevent the muscle from tightening up or shortening while in motion. This can be damaging to your heath as well as significantly decreasing the range of your movements. Static stretches are stretches where you hold still, you should try and do as regularly as you can if you want to gently increase your flexibility. Try and hold each stretch for at least 10 seconds, and no more than 30 seconds,. It's also important that you stretch all of the muscle groups before and after you have worked out. Finally and most importantly, a stretch is not a suitable warm up before physical activity! Warm up *before* you stretch. A good way to do this is to run on the spot for 60 seconds. If you don't warm up the muscle before you stretch, then you run the risk of damaging the filaments and the muscle itself. Here are four simple stretches to try:

Hamstring Stretch:

Put both of your feet together. Bend both of your knees and extend one leg forward, while keeping the other leg bent. Place your hands on the top of your right thigh and lean forward from the hips. Make sure that you keep your abdominal muscles tight and hold for about fifteen seconds. To enhance this stretch, raise the toes of your extended leg. Now repeat with the opposite leg.

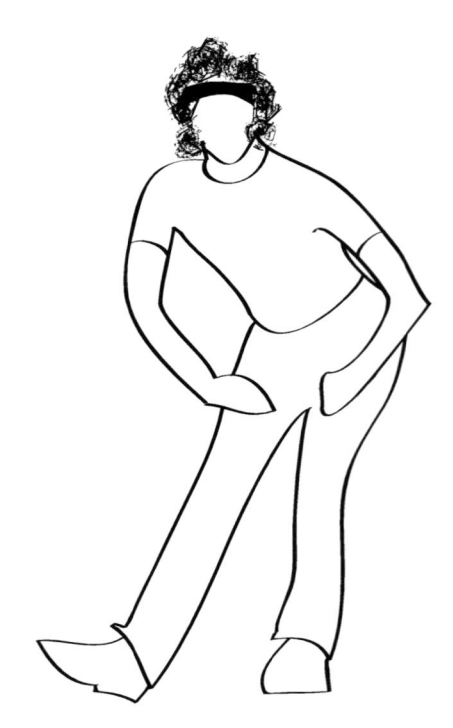

Front Thigh Stretch

You might want to get some stable support (like a chair or the side of a table). Start with your feet together and shift your weight onto one of your legs and soften the knee slightly. Raise the opposite leg (foot) up, toward your buttocks. Take hold of your ankle. Make sure that you keep your abdominal muscles tight and your knee facing the floor as well as your pelvis aligned and straight underneath you. Hold for 15 seconds and then repeat with the other leg.

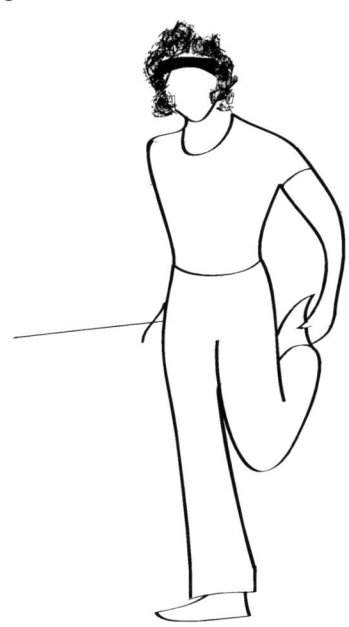

Calf stretch

Take a chair, or a stable support (like a table). Step forward with your back leg straight, in line with your back and your front leg bent at the knee. Make sure that the back leg is completely straight with your heel pressed against the floor completely and that your hips are aligned forward too. Your toes should be facing forward and there should be a straight line from the top of your head, through your back and down your leg, to the floor.

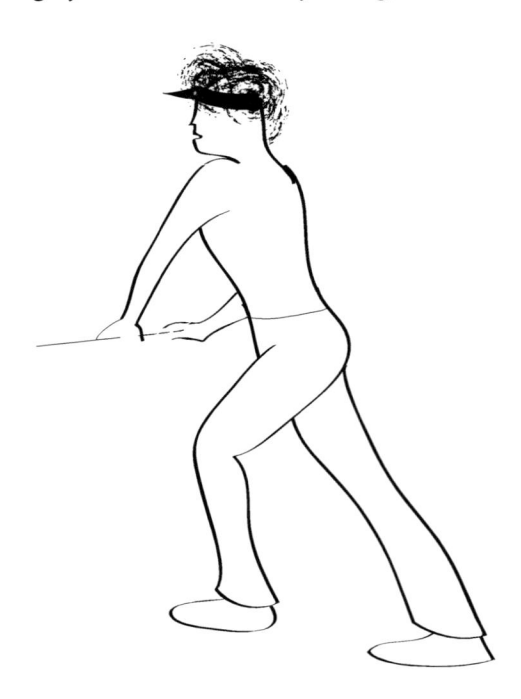

Dance & physical expression 171

Buttock Stretch

Hold your support and bend your supporting knee. Take the ankle of the opposite leg and bring it up in front of you and across the supporting leg. It should look like you're crossing your legs, in the air. Lean forward slightly from your waist, keeping your back straight, then relax and repeat with both legs.

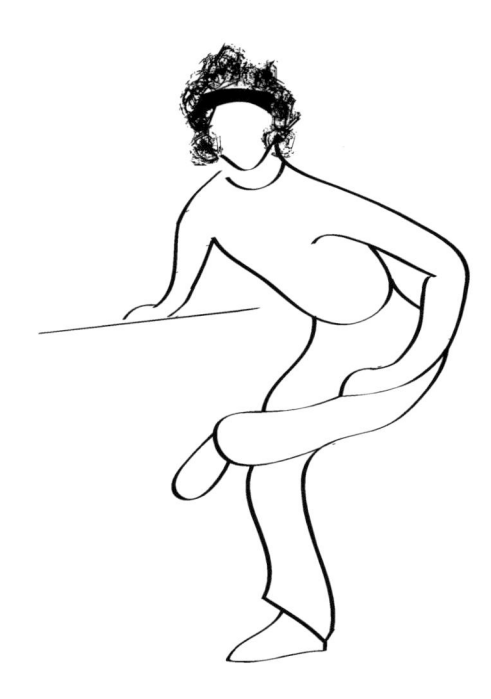

Some fun ways to keep toned!

Here are some of my favourite dance moves that are really fun and easy to do, that you can try at home!

Beyoncé style pump

- Make a fist with both hands
- Bend elbows and raise to chest level, knuckles facing inwards, elbows facing outwards
- Keep a slight gap between fists
- Pulse continuously as if lightly punching your fists away from your body
- Keep legs hip width apart and slightly bent

Pussycat doll prowl

- Bend both knees, step forward with your right leg, crossing your arms in front of your body, at the same time (lean slightly forward with your torso)
- Extend left leg to the left hand side, keeping weight on the right leg and opening both the arms at the same time to the side

- Repeat – this time stepping forward with the left leg out to the right and moving forward

The Thrust

- Do these moves in quick succession counting, "one, two, three, four." Thrust your chest forward and your shoulders back, at the same time, as far as they will go.
- Reverse the motion on the beat, bringing your shoulders forward and pulling your chest in.
- Vary the speed with the music, and add in a clap or a click of the fingers on the beat too!

Funky turn!

- Place your left leg in front of you, slightly bending the knee.
- At the same time, bring your arms up to chest level and swing them to the right. - Keep the back leg straight. In a swinging motion, pull your arms into your body, keeping your elbows up.
- Bring your right leg around and in a swinging motion propel your body around to the left…for a high energy funky spin!

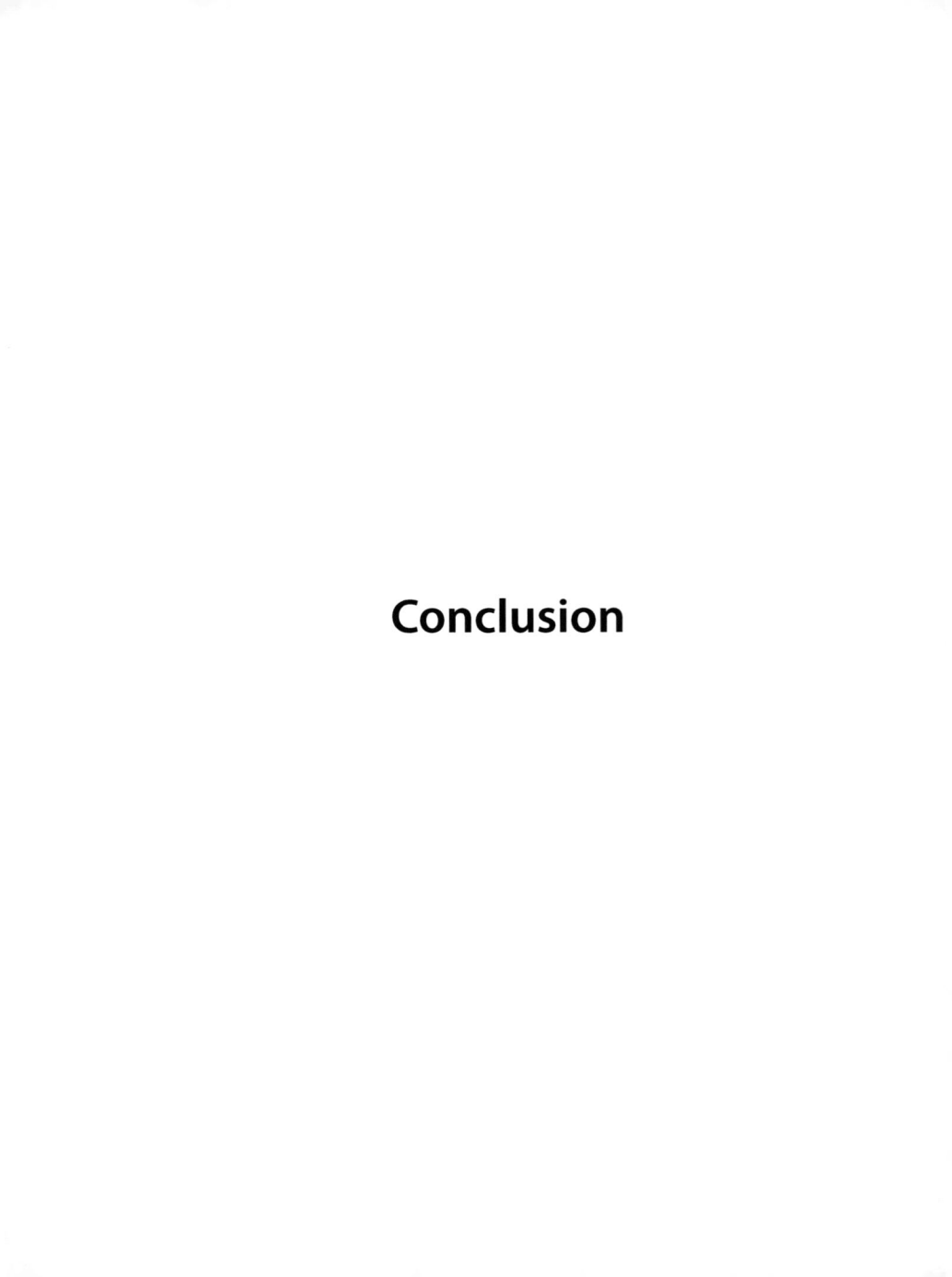

Conclusion

Conclusion: *acquiescing*

We've already determined that one day we will probably be old and grey and that we will probably ask ourselves some very interesting questions about the way in which we lived our lives. Did we let the world and the idiots around us determine the direction of OUR lives, dreams and goals? Or were we one of the few who did not acquiesce? Who did not compromise? Who had the courage and the sense to achieve whatever it was that we wanted to achieve that made us happy?

Unfortunately, the sad truth is that if any of us are one of those people, we are in the lonely minority. The majority will capitulate to societal pressure and the people around them. They will do it silently, without realising that they could have changed the situation at any time by speaking out. Some might have eventually realised that it didn't have to be that way…but it'll be too late by then. We only have one chance. To take what's ours, while we still can.

If we look to the various theological reference works we are generally given to believe that "faith can move mountains". In actuality this is just another convenient excuse for people who will do anything not to speak up, act and just follow the heart. Faith, belief, thoughts, opinion, imagination, visualisation, hallucination, waffle, talking a lot, praying a lot, making excuses, dreaming or even reading printed words on paper, without the key ingredient, have never moved a mountain…and never will.

If I personally ever felt the urge to relocate Everest (after becoming impatient with the current rate of lithospheric plate activity, I should add) I would plant down a few good old sticks of dynamite or alternatively…pick up a shovel and start digging quickly. No need for telekinesis or complicated theoretical excuses when simple action will do the job! Simple action is the key to success…it simply always has been.

Now, a conclusion!

What can I say that you don't already know? You are the number one expert in your life. So I ask you: How will you conclude? I'm curious…

Hopefully with some kind of action that will bring your dreams into reality…

I wish you success. Keep dancing

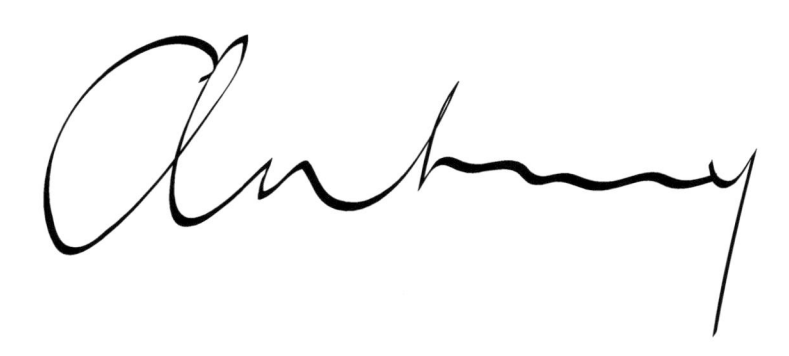

Acknowledgements

I would like to thank a few people who have been a great help to me while writing this book. First, Ryan Perera and family. Without you, I would not be here today and I thank you for everything. Sam Perera, thank you for your genius. Westley Harris, I'm very proud of you, thank you for always being there to pick me up. Man De Lev and Samir Suddle, thank you for your friendship, support and advice. Thank you for standing beside me. Thank you Mr Nick Mason and Pink Floyd, for your generosity and kindness. Extra special thanks to legendary Jeffrey Daniel! You are an amazing person. Thank you for supporting me and remaining so humble and kind. Shivy Gohil, thank you for your patience and amazing work, this project wouldn't be here if it wasn't for you and your talents! Thank you Raei for your friendship and for just being "the man". Philip Preiswerk and Philip-preiswerk.com…I thank you for your friendship, talent and support. Sidney, you are an amazing person, and I thank you for your friendship and inspiration and for being there. Pierluigi Gentile, thank you for your friendship and your amazing artistic talent. Thank you Sarah-Laure Estragnat for your support and friendship, you are a true artist. Thank you Claire and Punita, you two know the truth! I miss you. Debbie

Moore and Caleb Newman...I thank you for your support. Giles and Aina, two of the few with insight, I thank you. Mizuho, I haven't forgotten about you, thank you for your support. Special thanks to Dihan and FENEO.com...a true genius, I am grateful. Thank you to my Ozzy friends including the one and only Nick Schoonens! Thank you Yaro Starak, Renee, Phil Haddard, Jacqui and Lauren Heeney, I miss you Lauren. Extra special thanks to Otar "Get out the red" Campbell...I haven't forgotten about you and I miss you! Thank you Ryan, Westley, Richard, Marcia and Ashley. Thanks also to Amy and Liza, Dominic Berry, Tim Russell, Natasha Wright, Thea Thomson, Claire Singh, Claire "BEP", Vicky, Simon J Bailey...strike! (Legend), Rolfe Klement, Lil J, Lil Milk, Andrew Stone, Jagjeet Singh and family...I will never forget you (thank you Veteran for your wisdom), thank you Harish and family for your support, Nick Thornton, Maria Despina, Nadar, thank you Ernesto, Sarah Burkeman, Johnie Clayton, Richard Stanley, Dobs Vye, Cosima Somerset, Hamida and Akeel, thank you for your support, Liz Martin, Nicky Waterman, Drake (whatz up!), Sharon and everybody at Westfield, Daniel Miller, Robert Finegold, Elit Kane, Lauren Cochrane, Andrea Vakselj, Caroline Vaux, Claire Challinor, French Frederic, Jeff Eastman, Jernej Kosec, I miss you. Thank you "Lightcontrast" for giving me hope in the dark times.

Thank you Aidan, Mr C.L Amadain and June. Laura, Luke, Bron, Michelle, Louie, Michelle and the rest of the gang, I thank you. Thank you Rohin, Sanda Vidmar, Spela and Sarah Kirkham. Extra special thanks to Tick Tick Media, The Pirates and Pineapple Dance Studios Covent Garden, everybody at Vidal Sasson Covent Garden and the greatest stylist in the world: Pierluigi! Thank you Krishna, David Gamez, Johnathan Morris, "Shiv's dad", Mr Fossy, Ms Worswick and Mr Critchely (I hope you're proud…finally!). Thank you especially to Mr Cohen, Chris Oades and Mrs Franchesci… you all had a massively positive impact on me which I will never forget. Thank you Amato, my inspiration; Daniel, Flavia, Giulia, Tony (where are you?), Jay, Tarsilla, Daniella, Renato and Gustavo and the rest of the gang! Thank you Jean Michel Jarre and Aero Productions. Thank you Michael Tsarion, Henrik Palmgren, Francesc Marco, Remi, Thomas Jeffs, Davu, Michael Barnett, Drake and especially Michael Ang for getting me through. Thank you Jordan Maxwell and Alan Watt…I am eternally grateful. Thank you John Fisher and Mr D. Paul for your continuing support…

Finally, I'd like to especially thank Michael Jackson and Karen Faye for your kindness and support. Craig Murray and Nadira…my inspiration

Bibliography and Notes

Arden, Paul, It's Not How Good You Are, It's How Good You Want To Be, Phaidon Press, 2003

Bernstein, Richard, Dr.Bernstein's Diabetes Solution: Complete Guide to Achieving Normal Blood Sugars, Little, Brown & Company, 2004

Bilous, Dr. Rudy W, The British Medical Association Family Doctor Guide to Diabetes, Dorling Kindersley Publishers, 1999

Brzezinski, Zbigniew, Between Two Ages: America's Role in the Technetronic Era, Greenwood Press, 1982

Covey, Sean, 7 Habits of Highly Effective teenagers, Franklin Covey Co, 1998

Cummins, Stephen, Fibonacci Sequence, Xlibris Corporation, 2005

Dumas, Alexandre, The Count of Monte Cristo, Penguin Classics, republished 1997

Ellmann, Richard, Oscar Wilde, Vintage, 1988

Fistioc, Mihaela, the Beautiful Shape of the Good: Platonic and Pythagorean Themes in Kant's Critique of the Power of Judgment, Routledge, 2002

Franz, Marie-Louise von, Projection and Re-Collection in Jungian Psychology: Reflections of the Soul, Open Court Publishing Company, 1987

Freud, Sigmund, Leonardo Da Vinci and a Memory of His Childhood, W. W. Norton & Company, 1989

Freud, Sigmund, The Basic Writings of Sigmund Freud (Psychopathology of Everyday Life, the Interpretation of Dreams, and Three Contributions To the Theory of Sex), Modern Library, 1995

Gamez, David, What we can never know, Continuum, 2007

Guthrie, Kenneth Sylvan, the Pythagorean Sourcebook and Library: An Anthology of Ancient Writings Which Relate to Pythagoras and Pythagorean Philosophy, Phanes Press, 1987)

Hall, P, Manly, The secret teaching of all ages, J P Tarcher/ Penguin 2003 (original text published in 1928)

Hill, Napoleon, Think and Grow Rich, Ballantine Books, 1987

Howard Alex, Philosophy for Counselling and Psychotherapy: Pythagoras to Postmodernism, Palgrave Macmillan, 2000

Leitch, Adrienne, Dance: concise definitions of universal dance terms, Victoria, 2000

Livio, Mario, The Golden Ratio: The Story of PHI, the World's Most Astonishing Number, Broadway, 2003

Love, Roger and Frazier, Donna, Set Your Voice Free, Little Brown and Company 1999

Nelson, Portia, Autobiography in Five Short Chapters, There's a hole in my sidewalk, Beyond Words Publishing, 1993

Philips, Bill, Body for Life, Collins, 1999

Plato, the Republic, Penguin Books, 1955

Robinson, Ken, Out of Our Minds: Learning to be Creative, Capstone, 2001

Sobel, David, The Healthy Mind, Healthy Body Handbook, Time-Life Books, 1997

Shakespeare, William, Measure for Measure, Cambridge University Press, 1993

Tresniowski, Alex, When Life Gives You Lemons, McGraw Hill, 2000

Watts, Alan, The Book: On the Taboo Against Knowing Who You Are, Vintage, 1989

Watts, Alan, The Tao of Philosophy: The Edited Transcripts, Tuttle Publishing, 1999

Watts, Alan, Way of Liberation: Essays And Lectures On The Transformation Of The Self, Weatherhill, 1983

Wilde, Oscar, The Complete Works of Oscar Wilde: Volume 1, Poems and Poems in Prose, Oxford University Press, 2000

Anthony King, Part 3: Dance & physical expression; "Some fun ways to keep toned" originally published 2007 as "Anthony King's favourite dance moves" www.rimmellondon.com. Assistant choreographer: Lauren Heeney. Assitant Choreographer: Jacqui Heeney

Anthony King, Part 3: Dance & physical expression; "Control, placement and accuracy": Special thanks Jacqui Heeney: Artistic collaboration

Anthony King, Part 3: Dance & physical expression; "Learn the moonwalk". Originally published "Learn the moonwalk, by Anthony King": www.videojug.com / Sarah Birkham and "the moonwalk": "Anthony King's Thriller Dance Workout DVD"

Anthony King, Part 3: Dance & physical expression; "Learn the sideslide"; Originally published "Learn the Michael Jackson sideslide, by Anthony King": www.videojug.com /Sarah Birkham; and "The sideslide, by Anthony King": "Anthony King's Thriller Dance Workout DVD"

Special thanks to Shivy Gohil; graphic design and artwork on this book.

Special thanks to Mr Mohammed Nabulsi (MRPharmS) Member of the Royal Pharmaceutical society of Great Britain for being my nutritional advisor on this book.

DASH PHOTOGRAPHY

Design/artwork and illustrations by Shivraj Gohil
Photography by Dash Gohil

www.dashphotography.co.uk
www.shivyg.com
dash@dashphotography.co.uk

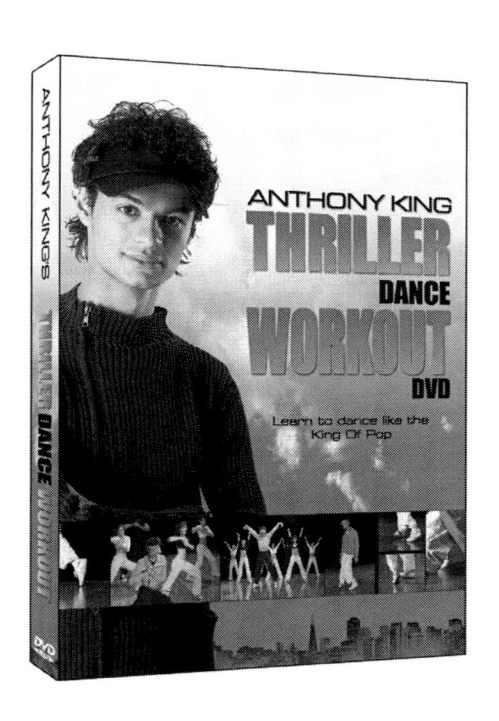

www.anthony-king.com

About the author

Anthony King is a young and successful choreographer and entertainer from London, England. He is a teacher at the world famous Pineapple Dance Studios where he teaches various styles including Commercial Pop and the acclaimed 'Michael Jackson Style Dance Class'. Anthony has been dancing and performing professionally since the age of 10 years old and has performed all over the world as a choreographer and artistic director. Anthony has choreographed Pink Floyd's Nick Mason; founding member of one of the world's biggest selling bands, who have sold over 100 million records. The biggest selling musical artist in the world, the King of Pop, Michael Jackson, has featured Anthony as BREAKING NEWS on his official website. His classes have been described by the 'THE SUN' newspaper as 'Hot!' 'Elle girl' magazine have featured his classes as the 'NEXT BIG THING'. He has been featured as a contributing writer for magazines including 'MORE MAGAZINE' as 'Celebrity dance tutor'. Anthony's class has featured on the hit show 'Bump n Grind' in which he starred as 'Booty camp' coach teaching the contestants some of his trademark moves and seriously putting them through their paces! Anthony is the 'Resident dance guru' for the fastest growing online expert video site videojug.com and has choreographed for the legendary BBC TV show Top of the Pops. He has been interviewed on the UK's biggest radio stations including BBC Radio 1, Capital FM and Choice FM. Rimmel London have featured Anthony as their 'celebrity choreographer' teaching his top 4 dance moves. Anthony has starred in and choreographed commercials for Sony PlayStation, Maverick Media, Warner Music and more. Described as an inspirational and unique teacher. He has held teambuilding events and dance workshops for some of the world's biggest companies including Red Bull, Proctor and Gamble and the Metro Newspaper group.

Anthony is available internationally for personal tuition, workshops, choreography and more:

www.anthony-king.com